Esthetic and Cosmetic Dentistry for Modern Dental Practice: Update 2011

Guest Editors

JOHN R. CALAMIA, DMD
RICHARD D. TRUSHKOWSKY, DDS
MARK S. WOLFF, DDS, PhD

DENTAL CLINICS OF NORTH AMERICA

www.dental.theclinics.com

April 2011 • Volume 55 • Number 2

SAUNDERS an imprint of ELSEVIER, Inc.

W.B. SAUNDERS COMPANY
A Division of Elsevier Inc.

1600 John F. Kennedy Boulevard • Suite 1800 • Philadelphia, Pennsylvania 19103-2899

http://www.dental.theclinics.com

DENTAL CLINICS OF NORTH AMERICA Volume 55, Number 2
April 2011 ISSN 0011-8532, ISBN-978-1-4557-0435-4

Editor: Donald Mumford; D.Mumford@elsevier.com

Dental Clinics of North America (ISSN 0011-8532) is published quarterly by Elsevier Inc., 360 Park Avenue South, New York, NY 10010-1710. Months of issue are January, April, July, and October. Business and Editorial Offices: 1600 John F. Kennedy Boulevard, Suite 1800, Philadelphia, PA 19103-2899. Periodicals postage paid at New York, NY and additional mailing offices. Subscription prices are $240.00 per year (domestic individuals), $420.00 per year (domestic institutions), $113.00 per year (domestic students/residents), $287.00 per year (Canadian individuals), $529.00 per year (Canadian institutions), $347.00 per year (international individuals), $529.00 per year (international institutions), and $170.00 per year (international and Canadian students/residents). International air speed delivery is included in all *Clinics* subscription prices. All prices are subject to change without notice. **POSTMASTER:** Send address changes to *Dental Clinics of North America*, Elsevier Health Sciences Division, Subscription Customer Service, 3251 Riverport Lane, Maryland Heights, MO 63043. **Customer Service (orders, claims, online, change of address): Elsevier Health Sciences Division, Subscription Customer Service, 3251 Riverport Lane, Maryland Heights, MO 63043. Tel: 1-800-654-2452 (U.S. and Canada). Fax: 314-447-8029. E-mail: journalscustomerservice-usa@elsevier.com (for print support); journalsonlinesupport-usa@elsevier.com (for online support).**

Reprints. For copies of 100 or more, of articles in this publication, please contact the Commercial Reprints Department, Elsevier Inc., 360 Park Avenue South, New York, NY 10010-1710. Tel.: 212-633-3812; Fax: 212-462-1935; E-mail: reprints@elsevier.com.

The *Dental Clinics of North America* is covered in *MEDLINE/PubMed (Index Medicus), Current Contents/Clinical Medicine, ISI/BIOMED* and *Clinahl*.

Printed and bound by CPI Group (UK) Ltd, Croydon, CR0 4YY

Transferred to Digital Print 2011

Contributors

GUEST EDITORS

JOHN R. CALAMIA, DMD
Professor; Director of Esthetic Dentistry; Director of the Esthetics Honors Program, Department of Cariology and Comprehensive Care, New York University College of Dentistry, New York, New York; Board of Directors, American Academy of Cosmetic Dentistry

RICHARD D. TRUSHKOWSKY, DDS
Associate Clinical Professor, Department of Cariology and Comprehensive Care; Associate Program Director of the International Program in Advanced Aesthetic Dentistry, New York University College of Dentistry, New York, New York

MARK S. WOLFF, DDS, PhD
Professor and Chair; Associate Dean, Department of Cariology and Comprehensive Care, New York University College of Dentistry, New York, New York

AUTHORS

ESTEVAM A. BONFANTE, DDS, MSc, PhD
Post-Doc Fellow, Department of Prosthodontics, UNIGRANRIO University, School of Dentistry, Rio de Janeiro, Brazil

LUIS BREA, DDS
Clinical Assistant Professor, International Program in Advanced Aesthetic Dentistry, Department of Cariology and Comprehensive Care, New York University College of Dentistry, New York, New York

JOHN R. CALAMIA, DMD
Professor; Director of Esthetic Dentistry; Director of the Esthetics Honors Program, Department of Cariology and Comprehensive Care, New York University College of Dentistry, New York, New York; Board of Directors, American Academy of Cosmetic Dentistry

RICARDO M. CARVALHO, DDS, PhD
Associate Professor, Department of Prosthodontics, University of São Paulo, Bauru School of Dentistry, Bauru, São Paulo, Brazil

GEORGE CISNEROS, DMD, MMSc
Professor and Chair of Orthodontics, Department of Orthodontics, New York University College of Dentistry, New York, New York

PAULO G. COELHO, DDS, PhD
Department of Biomaterials and Biomimetics, New York University College of Dentistry, New York, New York

STEVEN DAVID, DMD
Clinical Professor and Director, International Program in Advanced Aesthetic Dentistry, Department of Cariology and Comprehensive Care, New York University College of Dentistry, New York, New York

RENATA A. DIAS, DDS
Clinical Assistant Professor, Department of Prosthodontics, New York University, New York, New York

JONATHAN L. FERENCZ, DDS
Department of Prosthodontics, New York University College of Dentistry, New York, New York

STEFAN FICKL, DDS
Department of Periodontology, University of Würzburg, Würzburg, Germany

HUGH D. FLAX, DDS
President of the American Academy of Cosmetic Dentistry 2010–2011, Madison, Wisconsin; Private Practice, Atlanta, Georgia

RON GOODLIN, DDS, FAGD, AAACD
Director of Education for the Canadian Institute for Comprehensive Dental Education, Oakville; Smiles Dental, Private Practice, Aurora, Ontario, Canada

PETRA C. GUESS, DDS, Dr Med Dent
Department of Prosthodontics, Dental School, Albert-Ludwigs University, Freiburg, Germany

ERIK HAUPT, BA, AAACD
Lead Ceramist Haupt Dental Laboratory, Brea, California; Advisor, San Diego Advanced Study Group, Written Test Committee, AACD, Oragnathic Bioesthetic International Trained

MATTHIAS KRASSNIG, MD, DDS
Updent Dentists Vienna, Vienna, Austria

SO RAN KWON, DDS, MS, PhD
Department of Operative Dentistry, College of Dentistry, University of Iowa, Iowa City, Iowa

JONATHAN B. LEVINE, DMD
Program Director, Advanced Aesthetics Program, Department of Continuing Education, New York University College of Dentistry, New York, New York

YIMING LI, DDS, MSD, PhD
Professor of Restorative Dentistry and Director, Center for Dental Research, Loma Linda University School of Dentistry; Professor of Microbiology and Molecular Genetics, Loma Linda University School of Medicine, Loma Linda, California

MITCHELL LIPP, DDS
Clinical Associate Professor of Orthodontics, Department of Orthodontics, New York University College of Dentistry, New York, New York

ADRIANA P. MANSO, DDS, MSc, PhD
Courtesy Assistant Professor, Department of Operative Dentistry, University of Florida, College of Dentistry, Gainesville, Florida; Private Practice, Bauru, São Paulo, Brazil

JOE C. ONTIVEROS, DDS, MS
Head, Esthetic Dentistry; Associate Professor, Department of Restorative and
Biomaterials; and Director, Division of Biomaterials, Houston Center for Biomaterials and
Biomimetics, UT Health, The University of Texas Health Science Center at Houston Dental
Branch, Houston, Texas

ANABELLA OQUENDO, DDS
Clinical Instructor, International Program in Advanced Interdisciplinary Dentistry,
Department of Cariology and Comprehensive Care, New York University College of
Dentistry, New York, New York

THIAGO A. PEGORARO, DDS, PhD
Professor, Department of Prosthodontics, University Center, CESMAC, Farol, Maceio,
Alagoas, Brazil

GARY M. RADZ, DDS
Private Practice; Clinical Associate Professor, University of Colorado School of Dental
Medicine, Aurora, Colorado

STEFAN SCHULTHEIS, DDS, Dr Med Dent
Department of Prosthodontics, Dental School, Albert-Ludwigs University, Freiburg,
Germany

NELSON R.F.A. SILVA, DDS, MSc, PhD
Assistant Professor, Department of Prosthodontics, New York University College
of Dentistry, New York, New York

RICHARD D. TRUSHKOWSKY, DDS
Associate Clinical Professor, Department of Cariology and Comprehensive Care;
Associate Program Director of the International Program in Advanced Aesthetic Dentistry,
New York University College of Dentistry, New York, New York

JOHN F. WESTON, DDS, FAACD
Director Scripps Center for Dental Care, La Jolla, California; Board Member,
American Academy of Cosmetic Dentistry, Accredited Fellow of the American Academy
of Cosmetic Dentistry

MARK S. WOLFF, DDS, PhD
Professor and Chair; Associate Dean, Department of Cariology and Comprehensive Care,
New York University College of Dentistry, New York, New York

Contents

Even if a clinician possesses basic knowledge in esthetic dentistry and
clinical skills, many cases presenting in modern dental practices simply
cannot be restored to both the clinician's and the patient's expectations
without incorporating the perspectives and assistance of several dental
disciplines. Besides listening carefully to chief complaints, clinicians
must also be able to evaluate the patient's physical, biologic, and esthetic
needs. This article demonstrates the use of a smile evaluation form designed at New York University that assists in developing esthetic treatment
plans that might incorporate any and all dental specialties in a simple and
organized fashion.

The advent of digital photography allows the practitioner to show the patient the photographs immediately, to co-diagnose, and to work with the
patient chairside or in a consult room while showing the patient some simple imaging techniques, such as whitening the teeth, making the teeth look
longer, and showing the effects of orthodontics or veneers to get better
alignment and other factors of smile design and esthetic dentistry. This
article describes recommended digital dental photographic equipment,
how to produce the standard series of diagnostic dental photographs,
photographic assisted diagnosis and treatment planning including a discussion of anthropometrics and cephalometrics, and digital imaging
techniques.

This article discusses the possible methods available for whitening of a single discolored tooth. Treatment options can vary from restorative procedures such as crowns, veneers, or bonding to more conservative
bleaching treatments. The long-term success of the treatment is dictated
by proper diagnosis and treatment planning. The cause and severity of the
discoloration has to be carefully evaluated when planning for bleaching
options. The vitality of the pulp, presence and absence of symptoms,
and periapical pathoses usually determine whether an external or internal
bleaching approach will be considered.

> Crowded dentition is commonly found in the esthetic zone. Many forms of therapy can be used to treat the overlap of teeth caused by insufficient space within the dental arch. A careful analysis of patients with dental crowding is necessary to determine the most appropriate treatment of each individual case. Clinical considerations, advantages, disadvantages, and alternative treatment modalities for crowding dentition are discussed in this article and a clinical case is presented to illustrate the application of these techniques.

> Dental cements are designed to retain restorations, prefabricated or cast posts and cores, and appliances in a stable, and long-lasting position in the oral environment. Resin-based cements were developed to overcome drawbacks of nonresinous materials, including low strength, high solubility, and opacity. Successful cementation of esthetic restorations depends on appropriate treatment to the tooth substrate and intaglio surface of the restoration, which in turn, depends on the ceramic characteristics. A reliable resin cementation procedure can only be achieved if the operator is aware of the mechanisms involved to perform the cementation and material properties. This article addresses current knowledge of resin cementation concepts, exploring the bonding mechanisms that influence long-term clinical success of all-ceramic systems.

> Several all-ceramic systems have been developed in dentistry to meet the increased expectations of patients and dentists for highly aesthetic, biocompatible, and long-lasting restorations. However, early bulk fractures or chippings have led the research community to investigate the mechanical performance of the all-ceramic systems. This overview explores the current knowledge of monolithic and bilayer dental all-ceramic systems, addressing composition and processing mechanisms, laboratory and clinical performance, and possible future trends for all-ceramic materials.

> Porcelain laminate veneers (PLVs) provide the dentist and the patient with an opportunity to enhance the patient's smile in a minimally to virtually noninvasive manner. Today's PLV demonstrates excellent clinical performance and as materials and techniques have evolved, the PLV has become one of the most predictable, most esthetic, and least invasive modalities of treatment. This article explores the latest porcelain materials and their use in minimum thickness restoration.

High-quality aesthetic restorations that look great, function ideally, and last can only be predictably produced through implementation of excellent communication techniques and systems between the doctor and ceramist. With the availability of technology and the Internet, it is now easy to involve the laboratory via digital photographs. This article challenges one to begin including the laboratory early in the process and routinely use reliable techniques to transfer clinically significant information to the laboratory bench.

Laser technology has become preeminent in the evolution of appearance enhancements. Dentistry has seen a huge breakthrough with the introduction of a combination hard-soft tissue erbium wavelength. The conservative nature of this technique has created a firm footing in the antiaging trend that is spanning the globe. Among the many benefits of this technique are less invasive care and quicker healing responses. In this article, conservative laser and cosmetic modalities are discussed that allows a clinician to be more comfortable in buying a soft/hard tissue laser and also to more quickly become adept with implementing these techniques.

The selection of the best restoration for an endodontically treated tooth in the aesthetic zone depends on strength and the ability to recreate the form, function, and aesthetics of the natural tooth. The increased use of all-ceramic materials is a result of improved ceramic materials and adhesive systems. However, the advent of the current variety of translucent ceramic systems makes the shade of the abutment important in achieving the desired aesthetic outcome. This article discusses the different types of posts used in the restoration.

FORTHCOMING ISSUES

July 2011
Technological Advances in Dentistry
Harry Dym, DDS,
and Orrett Ogle, DDS,
Guest Editors

October 2011
Oral Surgery for the General Dentist
Harry Dym, DDS, and
Orrett Ogle, DDS,
Guest Editors

RECENT ISSUES

January 2011
**Contemporary Concepts in the Diagnosis
of Oral and Dental Disease**
Ira B. Lamster, DDS, MMSc,
Guest Editor

October 2010
Update of Dental Local Anesthesia
Paul A. Moore, DMD, PhD, MPH,
Elliot V. Hersh, DMD, MS, PhD,
and Sean G. Boynes, DMD, MS,
Guest Editors

July 2010
Current Concepts in Cariology
Douglas A. Young, DDS, MS, MBA,
Margherita Fontana, DDS, PhD,
and Mark S. Wolff, DDS, PhD,
Guest Editors

RELATED INTEREST

Oral and Maxillofacial Surgery Clinics of North America
February 2009 (Vol. 21, No. 1)
Complications of Cosmetic Facial Surgery
Joseph Niamtu III, DMD,
Guest Editor

THE CLINICS ARE NOW AVAILABLE ONLINE!

Access your subscription at:
www.theclinics.com

FORTHCOMING ISSUES

April 2011

Preface

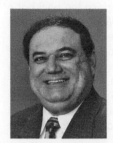 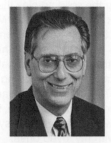 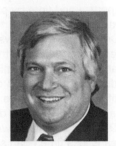

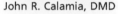

John R. Calamia, DMD   Richard D. Trushkowsky, DDS   Mark S. Wolff, DDS, PhD

Guest Editors

In April 2007 Elsevier/Saunders published an edition of *Dental Clinics of North America* entitled "Successful Esthetic and Cosmetic Dentistry for the Modern Dental Practice." As the senior editor of that issue, I selected authors and topics that would provide students of Esthetic Dentistry (whether they be generalists, specialists, seasoned practitioners, or recent graduates) with foundational knowledge in a clear and concise text to help them provide to their patients those often elective procedures requested in the modern-day practice of dentistry.

In the three years since that text has been available, I and my coeditors, Dr Mark Wolff and Dr Richard Simonsen, have received numerous accolades as to the relevance of those articles that, even today, provide still current and cutting edge information to readers, undoubtedly helping them to provide quality, long-lasting restorations for their patients. As originally predicted, some universities have used, with our blessings, the subjects covered in that text as a blueprint for their own esthetic curriculum, as modern day educators cater to the needs of our new generation of dental students at both the undergraduate and the postgraduate levels.

In this latest edition of *Dental Clinics of North America* I have again tried to not only update some of that foundational information in the articles on cements and new ceramics but I have also selected authors and topics that will provide the readership with evaluation and communicative skills that should allow for better diagnosis, better treatment planning, better case presentation, and better lab communication. This information, I am quite confident, will translate into better case outcomes that will provide functionally sound, physiologically healthy, esthetic results.

I have included case histories that encompass a large segment of the common esthetic needs of our patients including cases where multidisciplinary involvement is paramount to a successful outcome. Team dentistry is no longer ignored but is now the norm for many esthetic cases. Topics not covered in the original text such as comprehensive smile evaluation form, photography, temporization, and treatment of nonvital teeth have been included to round out a true esthetic curriculum. I am very hopeful that this edition will, like its predecessor, become a great reference source for those who want to provide the utmost in modern dental care. I am also hopeful that dental schools and other educational organizations and facilitators might consider this text as a solid reference guide to help update their own esthetic curriculum.

Dent Clin N Am 55 (2011) xiii–xiv
doi:10.1016/j.cden.2011.03.002
0011-8532/11/$ – see front matter © 2011 Elsevier Inc. All rights reserved.

dental.theclinics.com

I would be remiss if I did not express my sincere appreciation to the both nationally and internationally respected professionals who have, without financial rewards, given of their expertise and time by providing the solid articles that comprise the backbone of this text. I would also like to thank my coeditors, Dr Mark Wolff and new team member Dr Richard Trushkowsky, for their help and patience in editing as well as in their written contributions to this text. I would like to thank my parents, Mr Vincent Calamia and Ms Sina Calamia, for their unwavering belief that I could be both a good educator and a good dentist and then supporting me in my quest to enter this beautiful profession in the late 1970s. And finally I want to thank my family: my wife, Sonia Calamia, DDS, my daughter, Christine Calamia, DDS, and my son, Vincent Calamia, DDS, for putting up with me when I take on a busy project like this text, as it always means less time I can spend with my loved ones.

John R. Calamia, DMD
Department of Cariology and Comprehensive Care
New York University College of Dentistry
New York, NY 10010, USA

Board of Directors
American Academy of Cosmetic Dentistry
402 West Wilson Street
Madison, WI 53703, USA

Richard D. Trushkowsky, DDS
Department of Cariology and Comprehensive Care
New York University College of Dentistry
New York, NY 10010, USA

Mark S. Wolff, DDS, PhD
Department of Cariology and Comprehensive Care
New York University College of Dentistry
New York, NY 10010, USA

E-mail addresses:
jrc1@nyu.edu (J.R. Calamia)
ComposiDoc@aol.com (R.D. Trushkowsky)
mark.wolff@nyu.edu (M.S. Wolff)

Smile Design and Treatment Planning With the Help of a Comprehensive Esthetic Evaluation Form

John R. Calamia, DMD[a,b,*], Jonathan B. Levine, DMD[c],
Mitchell Lipp, DDS[d], George Cisneros, DMD, MMSc[d],
Mark S. Wolff, DDS, PhD[a]

KEYWORDS

• Smile • Design • Treatment planning • Evaluation form

In the modern practice of dentistry, it is no longer acceptable to just repair individual teeth. Increasingly more patients are demanding a final appearance that is not only physiologically and mechanically sound but also esthetically pleasing.[1] In addition to restoring and reconstructing the broken down dentition, bleaching, bonding, and veneering have opened the doors to a wide variety of elective dental treatments to enhance appearance, often reversing the visual signs of aging.[2,3] Understanding patient expectations is critical for clinicians to develop a treatment plan that is not only sound for the dental tissue but also esthetically pleasing. Often patients may not be able to identify their needs in anything more than short sentences stating their chief complaints. Clinicians must then decide whether the expectations can be met. If these expectations cannot be met, the case will likely fail.[4–6] Three simple questions, asked at the beginning of the Smile Evaluation Form, usually allow patients to express their needs clearly (**Fig. 1**).

[a] Department of Cariology and Comprehensive Care, New York University College of Dentistry, New York, NY 10010, USA
[b] American Academy of Cosmetic Dentistry, 402 West Wilson Street, Madison, WI 53703, USA
[c] Advanced Aesthetics Program, Department of Continuing Education, New York University College of Dentistry, 421 First Avenue, Rosenthal Clinic 1 W, New York, NY 10010, USA
[d] Department of Orthodontics, New York University College of Dentistry, 421 First Avenue, Clinic 5 S, New York, NY 10010, USA
* Corresponding author. DMD1 Amherst Place, Massapequa, NY 11758.
E-mail address: jrc1@nyu.edu

Dent Clin N Am 55 (2011) 187–209
doi:10.1016/j.cden.2011.01.012
0011-8532/11/$ – see front matter © 2011 Elsevier Inc. All rights reserved.

1. Are you happy with the way your teeth appear when you smille? **YES   NO   (circle one)**
2. If NO, what is it about your smile you would like to change?

Patients requests and expectations:

3. **Please Check Your Preferences:**
   O White Aligned Teeth
   O Natural Teeth with Slight Irregularities

Fig. 1. Questionnaire for patients to determine chief complaints.

If clinicians believe they have the experience and ability to meet the expectations, they must then carefully consider the patient in entirety.[7] This thorough evaluation must include a facial analysis, dental–facial analysis, and dental analysis, because each of these components and how they build on one another will provide the lattice structure for the finished case.

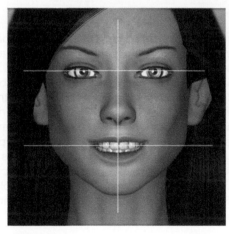

Lips

O Thick

O Medium

O Thin

Inter- Pupillary line
O Normal   O Slanted down   RT LT

Commissural line
O Normal   O Slanted down   RT LT   **Facial Analysis Frontal View**

Facial midline
O Normal   O Off to Patients   RT LT

Fig. 2. The first yellow horizontal line from the top is the interpupillary line. It passes through the center of the pupil of each eye. The horizontal line below this is called the commissural line, which passes through the corners where the upper and lower lips meet. These lines should normally be parallel to the incisal and occlusal planes of the patient's teeth. The thicknesses of the upper and lower lips are also noted and a description checked off. The need for possible lip enhancement or reduction also might be noted at this time. A vertical yellow line is drawn through the glabella (centered between the eyebrows), the tip of the nose, through the center of the philtrum, the center of Cupid's bow, and finally to the center of the chin. The resultant vertical line is the facial midline and is identified and analyzed as normal or curved. LT, left; RT, right.

FACIAL ANALYSIS
Frontal View

Facial analysis is checked at a conversational distance. The clinician uses a series of horizontal and vertical lines to determine the size and proportion of the face from chin to hairline and also the relationship of the patient's face and dentition in space (**Figs. 2–4**).

A profile view (**Fig. 5**) allows clinicians to visualize an important imaginary line called the *Rickett's E-plane*. This line drawn from the tip of the nose to the tip of the chin allows the profile of the patient to be evaluated by comparing the distance from this plane to the top and bottom lip. In the normal profile, the maxillary lip is approximately two times the distance (4 mm) as the lower lip to the E-plane.[8] A concave profile may call for a more prominent position of the maxillary anterior teeth with final restoration of the anterior teeth, whereas a more convex profile may require a more retruded position of the final restorations. Other imaginary lines form the nasal/labial line angle. In men the nasal-labial angle is generally 90° to 95°, whereas in women it is generally 100° to 105°.[9]

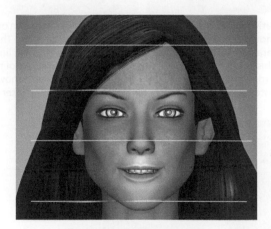

UFH -Upper Facial Height
LFH -Lower Facial Height
measured from [Sn - Me]
Sub-nasal (bottom of nose
meets upper lip) - menton
(bottom of the chin) landmarks

O WNL

O Excess L F H

O Deficient L F H

Fig. 3. The face is divided horizontally into three portions. The upper portion runs from the hairline to the top of the patient's eyebrows. The second portion runs from the eyebrows to the tip of the nose. The lower portion runs from the tip of the nose to the tip of the chin. This third portion is slightly wider than the upper two portions in a youthful patient with no occlusal wear and a normal vertical dimension. However, this portion may eventually shrink with age and severe wear (posterior bite collapse).

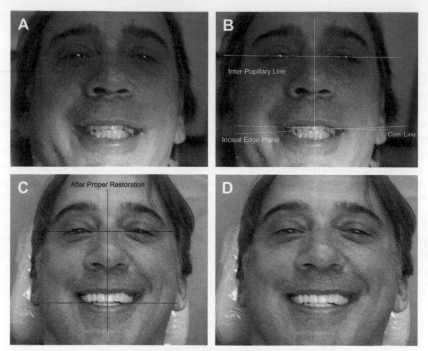

Fig. 4. (*A*) Pre-operative photo of a patient. (*B*) A patient with lines drawn on his before photo to simulate what should be observed using the smile evaluation form. The maxillary incisal edge should run parallel to the inter-pupillary and commissural (com) lines. Unfortunately as seen in this case this is not always true. In this patient the incisal edges of the maxillary anterior teeth run upwards from the patient's right to left. Figures *C* and *D* show the finished case with the restored anterior dentition incisal plane now parallel to the inter-pupillary line.

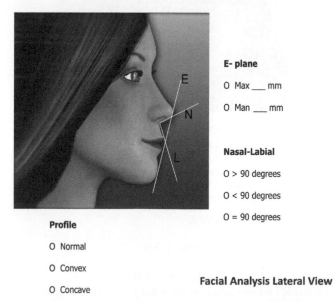

E- plane

O Max ___ mm

O Man ___ mm

Nasal-Labial

O > 90 degrees

O < 90 degrees

O = 90 degrees

Profile

O Normal

O Convex

O Concave

Facial Analysis Lateral View

Fig. 5. Profile view. Max__mm = distance measured from the maxillary lip to the E-Plane, (Avg. Caucasian −4, Avg. African American +4, [minus if concave facial form but plus if convex facial form]); Man__mm = distance measured from the mandibular lip to the E-Plane (Avg. Caucasian −2, Avg. African American +2, [minus if concave facial form but plus if convex facial form]).

Incisal and Occlusal Analysis

Next on the Smile Evaluation Form, the incisal and occlusal analysis is evaluated. This evaluation involves a good history that allows the clinician to diagnose whether habits have affected the occlusion, angulations, and buccal-lingual positioning of the teeth. If the clinician does not know the cause of an existing malocclusion/malposition, rebuilding the dentition may have short-lived outcomes. Overbite, overjet, space analysis, and classifications of occlusion and malocclusion should be evaluated carefully.

The functional assessment (**Fig. 6**A) occurs when a dental history is taken, and includes observations of the patient's swallowing and breathing during the initial visit. A thorough intraoral examination may show signs of bruxism and wear that could indicate incisal and occlusal disharmony. This evaluation also provides the best opportunity for clinicians to determine whether the facial and dental midlines are coincidental. If the maxillary or mandibular midlines deviate from the facial midline, this should be noted. Canting (a dental midline that is not parallel to the facial midline) has been shown to be even more discernable to patients and is considered more of a handicap

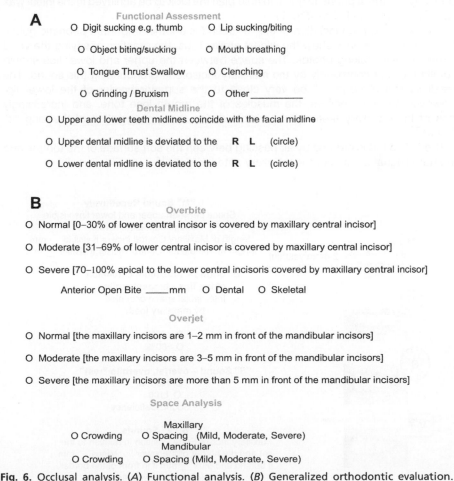

A

Functional Assessment

O Digit sucking e.g. thumb   O Lip sucking/biting

O Object biting/sucking   O Mouth breathing

O Tongue Thrust Swallow   O Clenching

O Grinding / Bruxism   O Other _____

Dental Midline

O Upper and lower teeth midlines coincide with the facial midline

O Upper dental midline is deviated to the   **R L**   (circle)

O Lower dental midline is deviated to the   **R L**   (circle)

B

Overbite

O Normal [0–30% of lower central incisor is covered by maxillary central incisor]

O Moderate [31–69% of lower central incisor is covered by maxillary central incisor]

O Severe [70–100% apical to the lower central incisoris covered by maxillary central incisor]

Anterior Open Bite ____mm   O Dental   O Skeletal

Overjet

O Normal [the maxillary incisors are 1–2 mm in front of the mandibular incisors]

O Moderate [the maxillary incisors are 3–5 mm in front of the mandibular incisors]

O Severe [the maxillary incisors are more than 5 mm in front of the mandibular incisors]

Space Analysis

Maxillary

O Crowding   O Spacing   (Mild, Moderate, Severe)

Mandibular

O Crowding   O Spacing (Mild, Moderate, Severe)

Fig. 6. Occlusal analysis. (*A*) Functional analysis. (*B*) Generalized orthodontic evaluation. L, left; R, right.

than dental midlines that are not coincidental but are at least parallel. A space analysis should also be categorized and noted.

In **Fig.** 6B, a generalized orthodontic evaluation (classification of occlusion or malocclusion) is noted. Orthodontic intervention may be considered a possible treatment adjunct or choice at this time.

Phonetic Analysis

In the 1950s, clinicians realized the importance of phonetics in determining denture teeth setup and appropriate anterior tooth position and length in relation to vertical dimension of occlusion.[10] A patient in physiologic rest position will normally have a 2- to 4-mm space between the upper and lower arch.[11] The minimum facial reveal of anterior teeth in this position for a youthful appearance has been identified as between 2 and 4 mm, depending on the sex of the individual (women generally show more tooth).[12]

The "m" sound allows a view of the rest position and the tooth reveal at this position. One may use this a phonetic guide to help plan the look to be achieved in the initial wax up of a well-planned case (**Fig. 7**).

The extended pronunciation of the "e" sound is another important phonetic guide. This sound will usually show the widest smile. Thus, the practice of saying the word "cheese" when taking photos. The space between the upper and lower lips should be filled almost completely by the maxillary incisors in pronouncing this sound. The Maxillary incisal edge will be very close to the superior border of the lower lip. However, as aging occurs, the muscles of the mouth lose tone, and increasingly less of the maxillary teeth will be visible during the pronunciation of the long "e" sound.[13]

The "s" sound is created by air passing between the soft surface of the tongue and the hard lingual surface of the maxillary anterior teeth.[14]

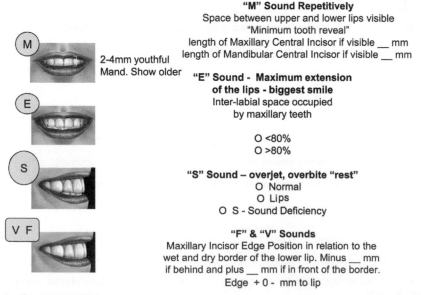

"M" Sound Repetitively
Space between upper and lower lips visible
"Minimum tooth reveal"
length of Maxillary Central Incisor if visible __ mm
length of Mandibular Central Incisor if visible __ mm

2-4mm youthful
Mand. Show older

**"E" Sound - Maximum extension
of the lips - biggest smile**
Inter-labial space occupied
by maxillary teeth

O <80%
O >80%

"S" Sound – overjet, overbite "rest"
O Normal
O Lips
O S - Sound Deficiency

"F" & "V" Sounds
Maxillary Incisor Edge Position in relation to the
wet and dry border of the lower lip. Minus __ mm
if behind and plus __ mm if in front of the border.
Edge + 0 - mm to lip

Fig. 7. Phonetic analysis.

Correct pronunciation of the "f" and "v" sounds is accomplished when the incisal edges of the maxillary anterior teeth come in light contact with the lower lip (vermilion border).[15] The incisal edges should be stationed directly over the line of demarcation between the wet and dry boarder of the lower lip. This mild contact allows a buildup of sufficient pressure for correct pronunciation.

A

Anterior Teeth Analysis
Mark any irregularities on the diagram for maxillary dentition

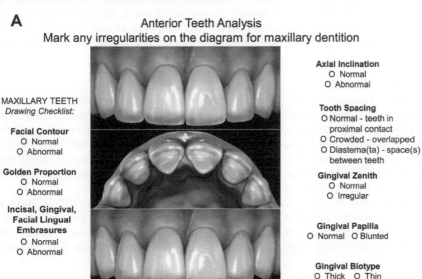

MAXILLARY TEETH
Drawing Checklist:

Facial Contour
O Normal
O Abnormal

Golden Proportion
O Normal
O Abnormal

Incisal, Gingival, Facial Lingual Embrasures
O Normal
O Abnormal

Axial Inclination
O Normal
O Abnormal

Tooth Spacing
O Normal - teeth in proximal contact
O Crowded - overlapped
O Diastema(ta) - space(s) between teeth

Gingival Zenith
O Normal
O Irregular

Gingival Papilla
O Normal   O Blunted

Gingival Biotype
O Thick   O Thin

B

Mark any irregularities on the diagram for mandibular dentition

Mandibular Teeth
Drawing Checklist:

Facial Contour
O Normal
O Abnormal

Proportion
O Normal
O Abnormal

Incisal, Gingival, Facial Lingual Embrasures
O Normal
O Abnormal

Axial Inclination
O Normal
O Abnormal

Tooth Spacing
O WNL
O Crowded
O Diastemata

Gingival Zenith
O Normal
O Irregular

Gingival Papilla
O Normal   O Blunted

Gingival Biotype
O Thick   O Thin "see through"

Non-vital tooth root – dark
Tetracycline stained teeth

Classification of Occlusion/Malocclusion

O normal
O Cl I Malocclusion
O Cl II Div 1
O Cl II Div 2
O Cl III

Fig. 8. (*A, B*) Dental analysis.

Dental Analysis

The maxillary and mandibular anterior dental analysis is made directly on the form using direct diagramming on the simple drawings or using the drawing checklist (**Fig. 8**). Facial contours that are irregular may be best seen in the incisal views, whereas golden proportion, incisal embrasures, axial inclination, tooth spacing, and gingival zeniths can be drawn directly on the facial views. Gingival biotype is also important to note, especially when deciding on the type of restoration to be used, because a thin biotype might require further gingival preparation to cover dark roots.

Dentofacial Analysis

A thorough dentofacial analysis is a critical component in determining the fine details of designing the restorations that will deliver the final esthetics of the case. Identifying the patient's horizontal and vertical components as either normal or needing improvement will help determine how the case should proceed (**Fig. 9**). After the Smile Evaluation Form has been used numerous times, the dentofacial analysis allows quick and accurate identification of problems. Any component that may require consultation with another discipline is easily identified and recorded.

Understanding the language of esthetics, a topic covered by Davis[16] in 2007, will help readers understand the diagrams on the Smile Evaluation Form.[15] This article explains the significance of important definitions such as lip line, midline, teeth exposed in physiologic rest position, and bilateral negative space. **Fig. 10** shows

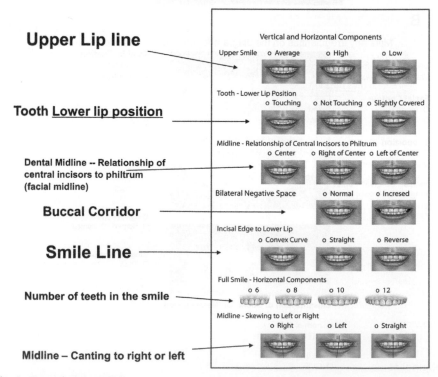

Fig. 9. Dentofacial analysis.

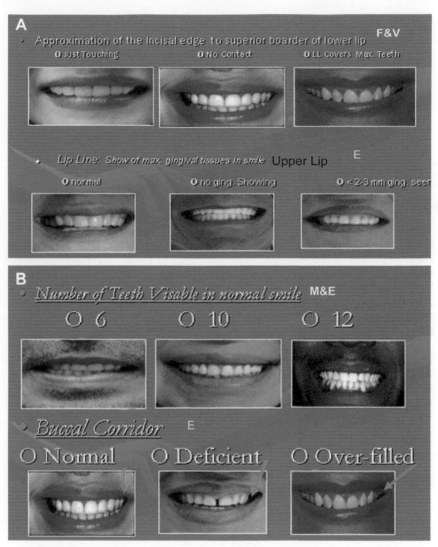

Fig. 10. Dentolabial analysis.

examples of normal and abnormal smiles. Most variations are present on the form to easily compare with the patient. In summary, the Smile Evaluation Form provides practitioners with a simple method of quickly notating the esthetic needs of the patient, and thereby will identify the disciplines that may need to be involved in a thorough treatment plan. This organized checklist provides clinicians with a goal, thereby allowing treatment sequencing to be planned better. The case presented in the next section was planned using this form and shows its usefulness (**Figs. 11–26**).

The following case will illustrate how the smile evaluation form can be used as an adjunct to collecting pertinent information needed to properly diagnose the patient's needs and help organize the patients final treatment plan.

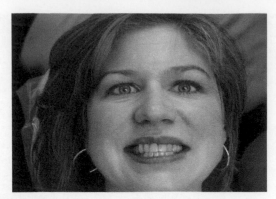

Fig. 11. Facial view.

Patient information
35-year-old Caucasian woman
Presented in March 2005
Very energetic and cheerful
Just bleached hair red in the past month (she is a natural brunette)
Reason for consultation
Chief Complaint: "One of my front left teeth has fractured on the edge and all
    my teeth look dull and are chipping."
History of the Chief Complaint: Fractured incisal edge tooth #10. No pain or sensi-
    tivity, but patient states that it feels "sharp and uncomfortable."
Initial consultation
Diagnosis and prevention
    Comprehensive history and examination
    Pulpal sensitivity testing
    Intraoral and extraoral photographs
    Diagnostic casts and mount
    Diagnostic wax-up

Intraoral Examination
Soft Tissue

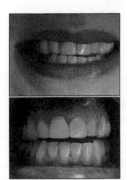

- Lips:
    - WNL
- Labial and Buccal Mucosa:
    - WNL
- Palate and Pharynx:
    - WNL
- Tongue:
    - WNL
- Floor of Mouth:
    - WNL
- Saliva:
    - WNL
- Breath Odor:
    - Slight halitosis
      food lodged in gingival
      embrasures

Fig. 12. Embrasures, incisal, gingival, facial, and lingual have been altered from existing bonding.

Maxillary Region

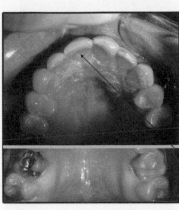

- - Composite Bonding
  Facial of Max. and Mand.
  Anterior Teeth
  #'s 5-13
  and #'s 22-27
  (3 yrs. old)

- - MO, OL Amalgam #3

- - O Composite #2, 12, 15,

- - MO, OL Composite #14

NB Dark stains of Tetracycline

Fig. 13. Incisal/occlusal view provides excellent view of the modified facial and lingual embrasures. Also noted are the dark tetracycline stains that are masked by excessive composite on the facial surfaces.

Mandibular Region

- -#18   O Composite
- - #19   MOD Comp. and
  B Amalgam Fillings

- - #30 RCT, Post ,Core,
  Crown (PFM)

- - #31 Occlusal Amalgam
  Filling
  (Margins slightly
  discolored)

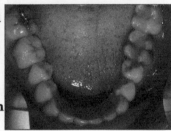

Fig. 14. Mandibular involvement of less concern.

Right Buccal View

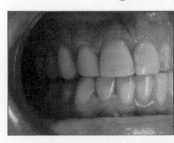
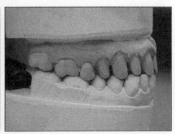

- #1, 32 missing
- Class I molar relationship
- Class I canine occlusion

Fig. 15. Occlusion is fairly stable on right side.

Right Periapicals and Bite Wings

- #2 Occlusal Comp. filling

- #3 MO, OL Amal. Fillings

- #30 RCT, P+C , PFM Cr.

- #31 O AMAL. filling

- Generalized bone loss slight WNL for 35 yr. old

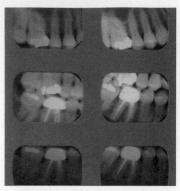

Fig. 16. Radiographic examination of right side normal with minor restorations present.

Left Buccal Region

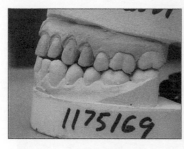 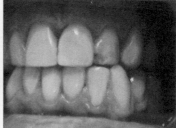

- Class I canine occlusion

- Class I molar occlusion

Fig. 17. Occlusion on left side.

Left Periapicals and Bite Wings

- #12 O Composite

- #18 with Class II MO Composite restoration

- #19 MOD Composite Restoration and B pit restoration Amalgam

- #20 Mesial pit filled with Amalgam DO Composite restoration

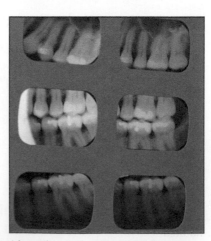

Fig. 18. Radiographic examination of left side with minor restorations present.

Orthodontic Evaluation

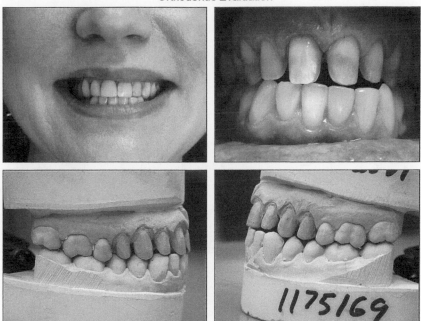

Fig. 19. Incisal edge shows distal shift #23.

    Oral hygiene Instruction
    Specialty consults: orthodontic and restorative
    Nutritional counseling
Medical history
Surgeries: None
Allergies: Penicillin
History of tetracycline use as a child
Social history
Single

Rotated Teeth

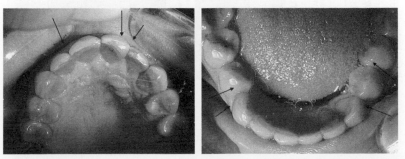

Fig. 20. Rotated teeth are identified. They have been treated with composite of differing thicknesses in order to improve the incisal appearance of the arch form.

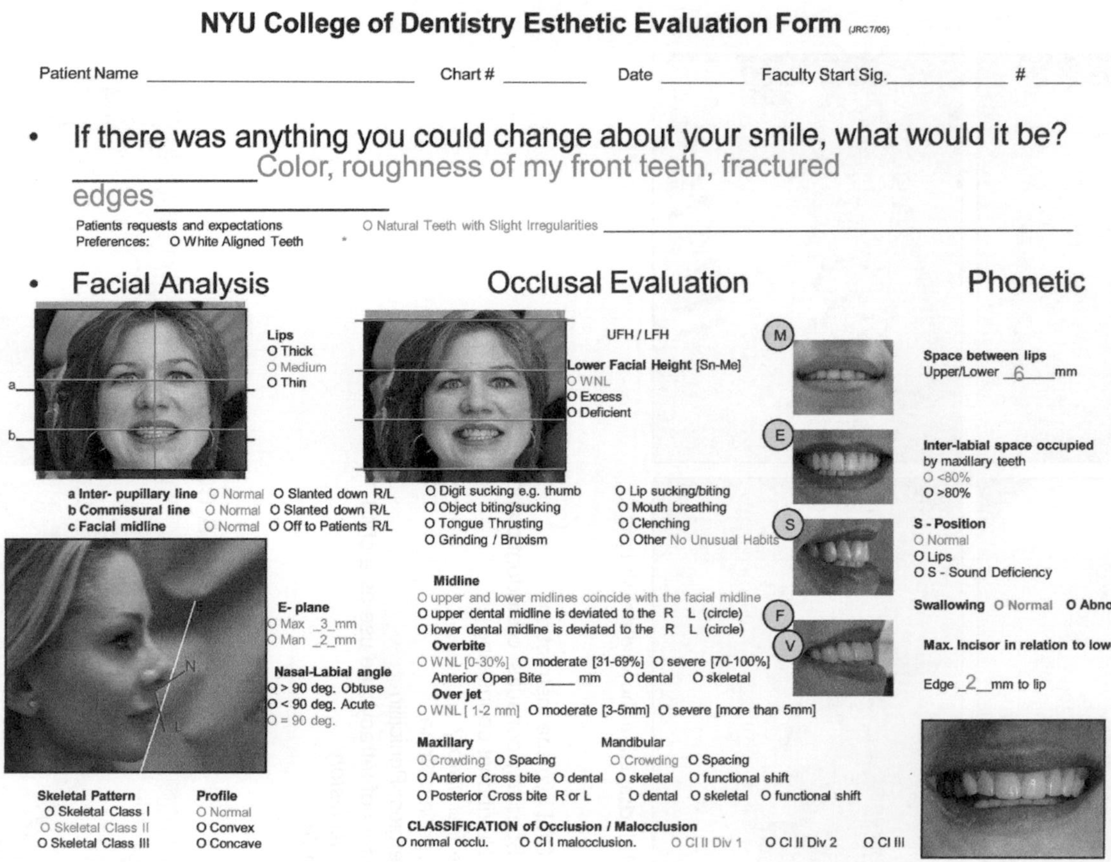

NYU College of Dentistry Esthetic Evaluation Form (JRC7/05)

Patient Name _____ Chart # _____ Date _____ Faculty Start Sig. _____ # _____

- If there was anything you could change about your smile, what would it be?
  Color, roughness of my front teeth, fractured edges

Patients requests and expectations   O Natural Teeth with Slight Irregularities
Preferences: O White Aligned Teeth

Facial Analysis

a Inter- pupillary line   O Normal   O Slanted down R/L
b Commissural line   O Normal   O Slanted down R/L
c Facial midline   O Normal   O Off to Patients R/L

Lips
O Thick
O Medium
O Thin

E- plane
O Max _3_ mm
O Man _2_ mm

Nasal-Labial angle
O > 90 deg. Obtuse
O < 90 deg. Acute
O = 90 deg.

Skeletal Pattern
O Skeletal Class I
O Skeletal Class II
O Skeletal Class III

Profile
O Normal
O Convex
O Concave

Occlusal Evaluation

UFH / LFH

Lower Facial Height [Sn-Me]
O WNL
O Excess
O Deficient

O Digit sucking e.g. thumb   O Lip sucking/biting
O Object biting/sucking   O Mouth breathing
O Tongue Thrusting   O Clenching
O Grinding / Bruxism   O Other No Unusual Habits

Midline
O upper and lower midlines coincide with the facial midline
O upper dental midline is deviated to the R L (circle)
O lower dental midline is deviated to the R L (circle)
Overbite
O WNL [0-30%] O moderate [31-69%] O severe [70-100%]
Anterior Open Bite ____ mm   O dental   O skeletal
Over Jet
O WNL [1-2 mm] O moderate [3-5mm] O severe [more than 5mm]

Maxillary   **Mandibular**
O Crowding O Spacing   O Crowding O Spacing
O Anterior Cross bite O dental O skeletal   O functional shift
O Posterior Cross bite R or L O dental O skeletal O functional shift

CLASSIFICATION of Occlusion / Malocclusion
O normal occlu.   O Cl I malocclusion.   O Cl II Div 1   O Cl II Div 2   O Cl III

Phonetic

(M) (E) (S) (F) (V)

Space between lips
Upper/Lower _6_ mm

Inter-labial space occupied by maxillary teeth
O <80%
O >80%

S - Position
O Normal
O Lips
O S - Sound Deficiency

Swallowing O Normal O Abnormal

Max. Incisor in relation to lower lip
Edge _2_ mm to lip

Fig. 21. Completed Smile Evaluation Form with answers in blue.

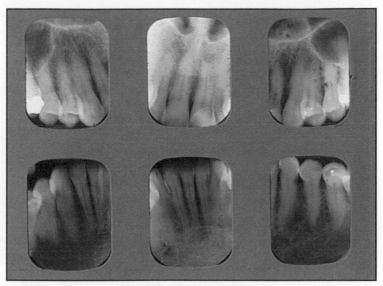

Fig. 22. Anterior radiographic examination normal.

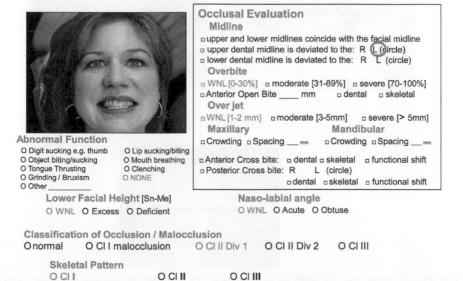

Occlusal Evaluation

  Midline
- □ upper and lower midlines coincide with the facial midline
- □ upper dental midline is deviated to the: R L (circle)
- □ lower dental midline is deviated to the: R L (circle)

  Overbite
- □ WNL [0-30%] □ moderate [31-69%] □ severe [70-100%]
- □ Anterior Open Bite ____ mm □ dental □ skeletal

  Over jet
- □ WNL [1-2 mm] □ moderate [3-5mm] □ severe [> 5mm]

Maxillary	**Mandibular**
□ Crowding □ Spacing ___ mm	□ Crowding □ Spacing ___ mm

- □ Anterior Cross bite: □ dental □ skeletal □ functional shift
- □ Posterior Cross bite: R   L (circle)
                       □ dental □ skeletal □ functional shift

Abnormal Function

O Digit sucking e.g. thumb	O Lip sucking/biting
O Object biting/sucking	O Mouth breathing
O Tongue Thrusting	O Clenching
O Grinding / Bruxism	O NONE
O Other _____	

Lower Facial Height [Sn-Me]   **Naso-labial angle**
  O WNL O Excess O Deficient   O WNL O Acute O Obtuse

Classification of Occlusion / Malocclusion
O normal   O Cl I malocclusion   O Cl II Div 1   O Cl II Div 2   O Cl III

  Skeletal Pattern
    O Cl I   O Cl II   O Cl III

Fig. 23. Close up of occlusal component of the patient evaluation.

Midline   - offset to the patients left

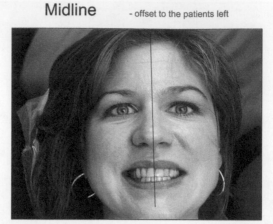

Fig. 24. Preoperative evaluation of the dental midline compared with the patient's facial midline. The dental midline is slightly offset to the patient's left in comparison to the facial midline.

A Smile Line – slightly concave
Does <u>not</u> follow the lower lip!

B Axial Inclination

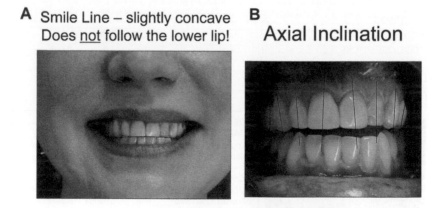

C Gingival Zeniths

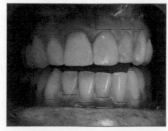

Fig. 25. (*A*) Smile line, (*B*) axial inclination, and (*C*) gingival zeniths are examined. The normal lip line hides minor gingival zenith discrepancies.

Restorative Considerations?

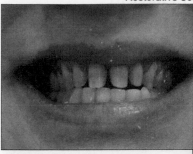

Location of Tetra. Bands !
Color of Bands !
Stump Shade !

Should Bleaching be done first?

Should the preparation be Deeper ?

Type of Porcelain USED?
Opaquer Added?

Type of Cements USED ?

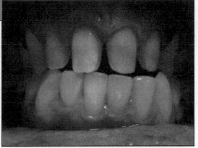

Fig. 26. Location of tetracycline (tetra) bands and their degree of darkness may have implications on depth of preparation and preferred material for final restoration.

Employed
Social drinker
Does not smoke
Dental-oral history
Last visit was 6 months before consultation
Mostly regular visits
Minor restorative work anterior (3 years ago)
   (composite bonding facial of maxillary and mandibular anterior teeth)
Extensive restorative work posterior
   MO, OL amalgam #3
   MO, OL composite #14
   MOD composite #19 with buccal amalgam pit
   O composite #2, #12, #15, and #17
   O amalgam #31
Root canal therapy, post, core, and crown (PFM) #31
Medications
Vitamin E
Extraoral examination
Appearance is well-groomed and neat
Skin, head, and neck: WNL
Muscles: WNL
Temporomandibular joint: WNL
Vitals
Blood pressure: 120/80
Heart rate: 67 beats per minute
Respiratory rate: 14 respirations per minute
Weight: 118 lb.

Porcelain Design

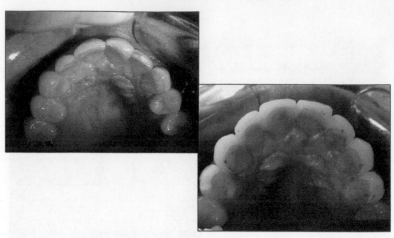

Fig. 27. Incisal view showing depth and finishing lines of the preparation design which in turn will affect arch form.

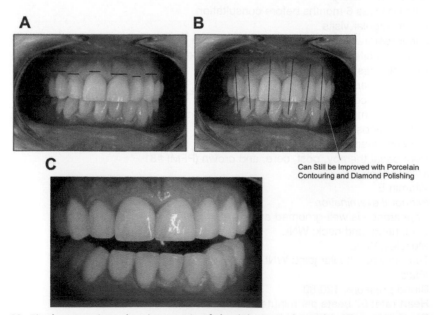

Can Still be Improved with Porcelain
Contouring and Diamond Polishing

Fig. 28. Final restorations showing repair of the (A) gingival zeniths, (B) axial inclination, and (C) smile line.

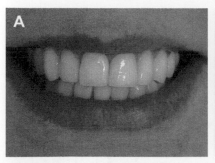

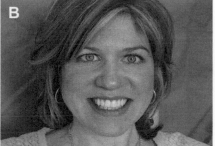

Fig. 29. (*A*) The dental and facial midlines are now coincidental. (*B*) Although the patient has red hair, a light shade of Vita B1 was selected. The literature has shown that individuals with red hair generally have yellow-orange tint in their natural dentition.

Problem list derived from Smile Evaluation Form
Occlusion
Possible labial shift
Oral hygiene
Fair to good
Esthetics
Generalized tooth discoloration (origin: tetracycline)
Anterior bonding: Overcontoured, discolored, and cracking
Plaque accumulation on rough surface of old bonding
Diagnosis
Broken down bonding

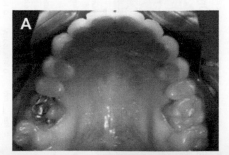

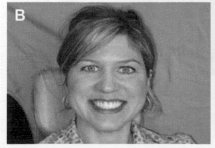

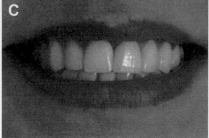

Fig. 30. (*A–C*) One-year recall of restorations. Patient changed to blond highlights in her hair.

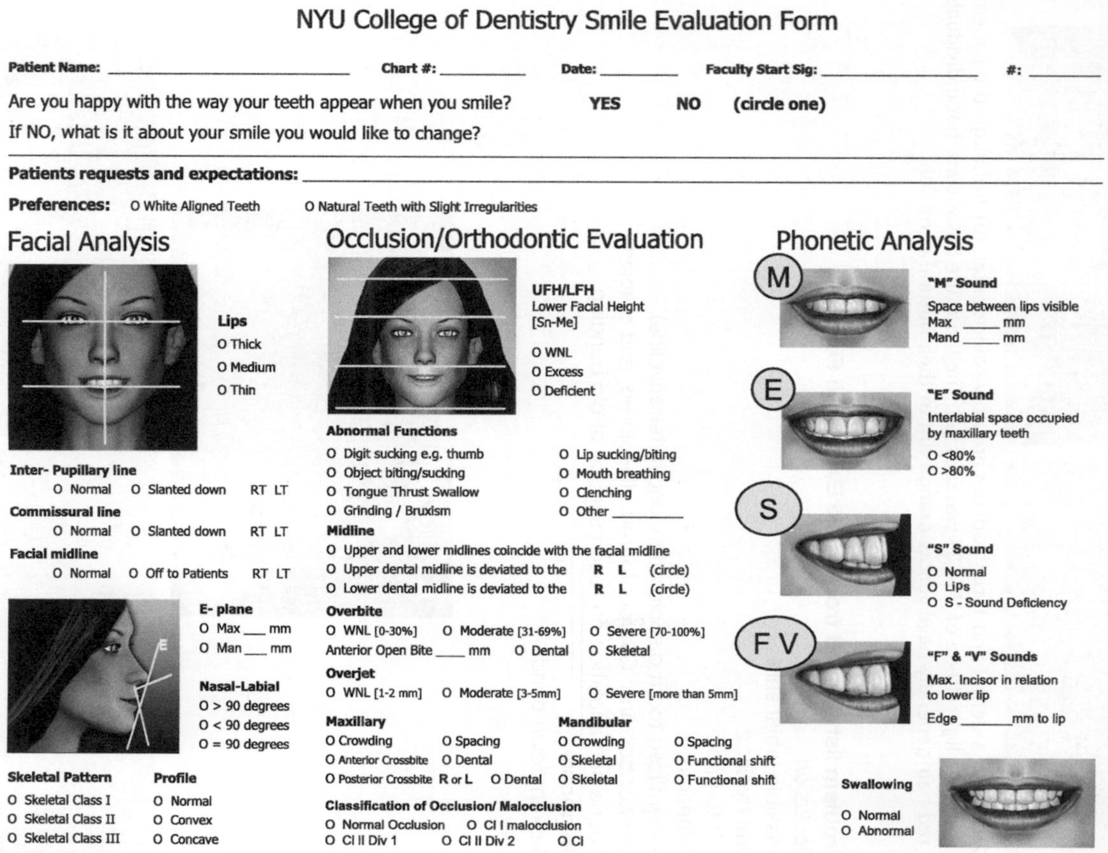

NYU College of Dentistry Smile Evaluation Form

Patient Name: _____   **Chart #:** _____   **Date:** _____   **Faculty Start Sig:** _____   **#:** _____

Are you happy with the way your teeth appear when you smile?   **YES   NO**   (circle one)

If NO, what is it about your smile you would like to change?

Patients requests and expectations:

Preferences: O White Aligned Teeth   O Natural Teeth with Slight Irregularities

Facial Analysis

Lips
O Thick
O Medium
O Thin

Inter- Pupillary line
O Normal   O Slanted down   RT LT

Commissural line
O Normal   O Slanted down   RT LT

Facial midline
O Normal   O Off to Patients   RT LT

E- plane
O Max _____ mm
O Man _____ mm

Nasal-Labial
O > 90 degrees
O < 90 degrees
O = 90 degrees

Skeletal Pattern
O Skeletal Class I
O Skeletal Class II
O Skeletal Class III

Profile
O Normal
O Convex
O Concave

Occlusion/Orthodontic Evaluation

UFH/LFH
Lower Facial Height [Sn-Me]
O WNL
O Excess
O Deficient

Abnormal Functions
O Digit sucking e.g. thumb
O Object biting/sucking
O Tongue Thrust Swallow
O Grinding / Bruxism

O Lip sucking/biting
O Mouth breathing
O Clenching
O Other _____

Midline
O Upper and lower midlines coincide with the facial midline
O Upper dental midline is deviated to the   R L (circle)
O Lower dental midline is deviated to the   R L (circle)

Overbite
O WNL [0-30%]   O Moderate [31-69%]   O Severe [70-100%]
Anterior Open Bite _____ mm   O Dental   O Skeletal

Overjet
O WNL [1-2 mm]   O Moderate [3-5mm]   O Severe [more than 5mm]

Maxillary
O Crowding   O Spacing
O Anterior Crossbite O Dental
O Posterior Crossbite R or L O Dental

Mandibular
O Crowding   O Spacing
O Skeletal   O Functional shift
O Skeletal   O Functional shift

Classification of Occlusion/ Malocclusion
O Normal Occlusion   O Cl I malocclusion
O Cl II Div 1   O Cl II Div 2   O Cl

Phonetic Analysis

"M" Sound
Space between lips visible
Max _____ mm
Mand _____ mm

(M)

"E" Sound
Interlabial space occupied by maxillary teeth
O <80%
O >80%

(E)

"S" Sound
O Normal
O Lips
O S - Sound Deficiency

(S)

"F" & "V" Sounds
Max. Incisor in relation to lower lip
Edge _____ mm to lip

(F V)

Swallowing
O Normal
O Abnormal

Fig. 31. Smile Evaluation Form side A.

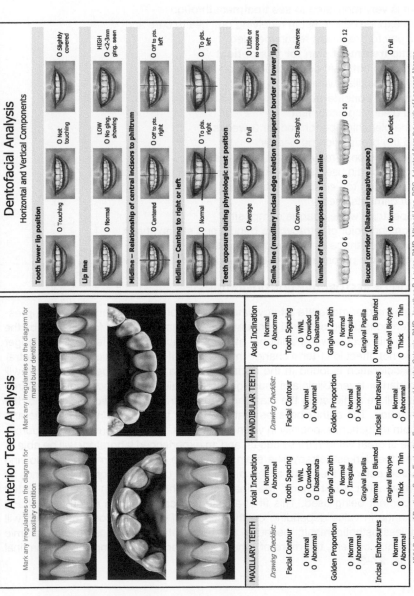

Fig. 32. Smile Evaluation Form side B.

The following text is within the figure image:

Dentofacial Analysis
Horizontal and Vertical Components

Tooth lower lip position
- O Touching
- O Not touching
- O Slightly covered

Lip line
- O Normal
- LOW O No ging. showing
- HIGH O <2-3mm ging. seen

Midline — Relationship of central incisors to philtrum
- O Centered
- O Off to pts. right
- O Off to pts. left

Midline — Canting to right or left
- O Normal
- O To pts. right
- O To pts. left

Teeth exposure during physiologic rest position
- O Average
- O Full
- O Little or no exposure

Smile line (maxillary incisal edge relation to superior border of lower lip)
- O Convex
- O Straight
- O Reverse

Number of teeth exposed in a full smile
- O 6
- O 8
- O 10
- O 12

Buccal corridor (bilateral negative space)
- O Normal
- O Defect
- O Full

Anterior Teeth Analysis

Mark any irregularities on the diagram for maxillary dentition

Mark any irregularities on the diagram for mandibular dentition

MAXILLARY TEETH

Drawing Checklist:

Facial Contour
- O Normal
- O Abnormal

Golden Proportion
- O Normal
- O Abnormal

Incisal Embrasures
- O Normal O Blunted

Gingival Biotype
- O Thick O Thin

Axial Inclination
- O Normal
- O Abnormal

Tooth Spacing
- O WNL
- O Crowded
- O Diastemata

Gingival Zenith
- O Normal
- O Irregular

Gingival Papilla
- O Normal O Blunted

MANDIBULAR TEETH

Drawing Checklist:

Facial Contour
- O Normal
- O Abnormal

Golden Proportion
- O Normal
- O Abnormal

Incisal Embrasures
- O Normal
- O Abnormal

Axial Inclination
- O Normal
- O Abnormal

Tooth Spacing
- O WNL
- O Crowded
- O Diastemata

Gingival Zenith
- O Normal
- O Irregular

Gingival Biotype
- O Thick O Thin

NYU College of Dentistry Smile Evaluation Form designed by John Calamia, DMD, Jonathan B. Levine, DMD, Mitchell Lipp, DDS. Adapted from the work of Leonard Abrams, 255 South Seventeenth Street, Philadelphia, PA 19103 1987 and Dr. Mauro Fradeani Esthetic Rehabilitation in Fixed Prosthodontics Quintessence Publishing Co. Inc Carol Stream, IL 2004 Jonathan B. Levine, DMD GoSMILE Aesthetics 923 5th Avenue, New York, NY 10021

Generalized mild gingivitis from rough and overcontoured
   bonded surfaces
Slightly compromised function
Prognosis
Good to excellent
Patient is very motivated to see treatment through
Patient expressed interest in receiving oral health care and
   will pay for treatment recommended
Realistic treatment plan for this patient
Patient does not want orthodontic option and
   prefers maxillary veneers
Restorative considerations
Should bleaching occur first
At-home bleaching performed for 3 weeks
Should the preparation be deeper
Less preparation is required in a young patient
Type of porcelain used/should opaque be added to this porcelain
Opaque added to Feldspathic porcelain
Type of cements used
TPH Spectrum white opaque composite
Location and color of tetracycline bands, and stump shade
Stump shade (shade of the prepared tooth) and a digital
   photo of the prepared teeth sent to laboratory technician.

DISCUSSION OF RESTORATIVE CONSIDERATIONS

Bleaching of mild or moderate tetracycline cases before preparation and final impression is often considered practical because it may negate the need for masking by the ceramist. If this occurs with traditional at-home bleaching, the effect will last longer and should not affect long-term change in final color of the restoration. Because tetracycline discoloration is found in the dentin layer of a tooth, deeper preparation will expose a darker layer. Clinicians must gauge the value of this reduction compared with what will be achieved in the masking resulting from the added thickness of the final restoration. The author believes that it is better to do more in the ceramic and less in tooth reduction, especially in younger patients. Using a more opacious porcelain can be of great value in these cases, and an experienced laboratory will be able to mask even the darkest tetracycline stains if they are given a stump shade showing the prepared color of the tooth and a digital image of the location of the bands of discoloration. After a last check, the final color of the restoration may be adjusted with the cement being used. This final adjustment can affect as much as a shade or two change in value depending on the degree of opacity introduced, which will impart a less-esthetic result, because the closer the clinician is to the ceramic with an opaque cement, the more of a headlight effect may be imparted to the final shade (**Figs. 27–30**).

SUMMARY

The authors have introduced a Smile Evaluation Form to help clinicians handle difficult esthetic cases (**Figs. 31** and **32**). This form is currently in use in the New York University College of Dentistry's clinics and is taught in the first- and second-year preclinical courses. This form is considered modifiable and the authors are open to critical suggestions for improvement.

ACKNOWLEDGMENTS

The authors would like to acknowledge the pioneering work performed in this field of evaluation forms by Dr Leonard Abrams, Dr Jeffrey Morley, Dr James Eubank, Dr Mauro Fradeani,[17] and Dr Jonathan Levine.

REFERENCES

1. Spear FM, Kokich VG. A multidisciplinary approach to esthetic dentistry, 51. Dent Clin North Am; 2007. p. 487–505.
2. Dzierzak J. Restoring the aging dentition. Curr Opin Cosmet Dent 1995;41–4.
3. Morley J. The role of cosmetic dentistry in restoring a youthful appearance. J Am Dent Assoc 1999;130:1166–72.
4. Goldstein RE. Study of the need for esthetics in dentistry. J Prosthet Dent 1969; 21:589–98.
5. Goldstein RE, Lancaster JS. Survey of patient attitudes toward current esthetic procedures. J Prosthet Dent 1984;52:775–80.
6. Feeley RT. Cosmetics and the esthetic patient and laboratory communication. Oral Health 1995;85:9–14.
7. Morley J, Eubank J. Macro-esthetic element of smile design. J Am Dent Assoc 2001;132:39–45.
8. Ricketts RM. Planning treatment on the basis of facial pattern and an estimate of its growth. Angle Orthod 1957;27:14–37.
9. Levine JB. Esthetic diagnosis. In: current concepts in cosmetic dentistry. Chicago: Quintessence Publishing; 1994. 9–17.
10. Pound E. Esthetic dentures and their phonetic values. J Prosthet Dent 1951;2: 98–112.
11. Rugh JD, Drago CJ, Barghi N. Comparison of electromyographic and phonetic measurements of vertical rest position [abstract]. J Dent Res 1979;58(Suppl):316.
12. Vig RG, Brundo GC. The kinetics of anterior tooth display. J Prosthet Dent 1978; 39:502–54.
13. Hammond RJ, Beder OE. Increased vertical dimension and speech articulation errors. J Prosthet Dent 1984;52(3):401–46.
14. Spear FM. Fundamental occlusal therapy of occlusion. In: McNeill C, editor. Science and practice of occlusion. Chicago: Quintessence; 1997. p. 421–34.
15. Dawson PE. Restoring upper anterior teeth. In: Dawson PE, editor. Evaluation, diagnosis, and treatment problems. 2nd edition. St. Louis (MO): Mosby; 1989. p. 325.
16. Davis NC. Smile design. Dent Clin North Am 2007;51:299–318.
17. Fradeani M. Esthetic analysis, a systematic approach to prosthetic treatment. Chicago: Quintessence; 2004.

Photographic-Assisted Diagnosis and Treatment Planning

Ron Goodlin, DDS

KEYWORDS

- Photographic-assisted diagnosis
- Photographic-assisted treatment planning
- Standard series of dental photographs
- Dental photographic equipment

Standard of practice is defined as the best most often used technique, method, process, or activity that is believed to be more effective at delivering a particular outcome than any other technique, method, process, and so forth. With proper processes, a desired outcome can be delivered with fewer problems and unforeseen complications in the most efficient and effective way of accomplishing a task, based on repeatable procedures that have proven themselves over time for large numbers of people. Standard of practice refers to the level of treatment that would be expected from a competent practitioner, and is readily accepted by most practitioners in that field.[1]

Digital dental photography is the standard of care, the standard of practice, and the best practice in esthetic dentistry.

Diagnosis and treatment planning of esthetic cases requires the use of photographs that are specifically designed to give the practitioner the information required to make that diagnosis and develop the treatment plan. Just as an orthodontist would never proceed without a cephalometric radiograph or a series of photographs, so to the "cosmetic dentist" should never proceed without a standard series of dental photographs specifically designed to assist in the diagnosis and treatment planning of the case.

Three important questions must be answered: (1) what photographs are required, (2) how do we take them, and (3) how do we interpret them to do the diagnosis and treatment planning required?

The standardization of clinical photographs was first described by this author in 1979[2] where the importance of standardization in views, magnification ratios, procedure, and lighting was discussed to enable the practitioner to compare photographic views before and after and between practitioners all over the world as the standard.

Smiles Dental, 15213 Yonge Street, Suite 6, Aurora, ON L4G 1L8, Canada
E-mail address: ron@smiledental.ca

Dent Clin N Am 55 (2011) 211–227
doi:10.1016/j.cden.2011.02.001
0011-8532/11/$ – see front matter © 2011 Elsevier Inc. All rights reserved.

dental.theclinics.com

This series has evolved to include more photographs beyond the basic series that was designed originally for orthodontic case comparison and has now grown to involve all forms of dentistry. It should be remembered that the standard series for a cosmetic dentist will be slightly different than for an orthodontist, or general dental practitioner. Each practitioner must determine what the correct number and views will be for the clinical purposes defined. The originally described standard intraoral photographic series included 2 extraoral views (face and profile views) and 5 intraoral views (retracted anterior, right and left lateral, and 2 occlusal views).

The original intent has not changed, as the usefulness of comparison of cases before and after will always be of great benefit. But as described, the uses have expanded such that every patient will have a complete set of photographic records before treatment and after treatment to defend litigation, to improve one's level of dental skill, to use for marketing, and of course to assist in diagnosis and treatment planning.

The advent of digital photography allows the practitioner to show the patient the photographs immediately, to co-diagnose, and to work with the patient chairside or in a consult room while showing the patient some simple imaging techniques, such as whitening the teeth, making the teeth look longer, and showing the effects of orthodontics or veneers to get better alignment and other factors of smile design and esthetic dentistry.

With progress in esthetic technique and understanding, we have come to learn other very important views to help assist the practitioner in diagnosis and treatment planning. The American Academy of Cosmetic Dentistry describes their required standard series of accreditation photographs to include a facial view, 3 smile views, 3 retracted views, 3 close-up views, and 2 occlusal views (**Fig. 1**).

Through the work of Spear,[3] and this author, additional views have been shown to have extreme importance in the evaluation of the maxillary incisal edge position (IEP), arguably the most important first step in the development of the new smile. These include the tooth shown at rest view, the incisal edge "VVVV" position, and the horizontal "VVVV" position to determine IEP and neutral zone horizontal position (**Fig. 2**).

EQUIPMENT REQUIREMENTS AND PHOTOGRAPHIC PRINCIPLES

Dental photography equipment should be part of the dental armamentarium.[4] It should always be available to the practitioner or staff and should therefore remain on the office premises at all times. The camera equipment you will use for digital dental photography is arguably completely different from your "at-home photography equipment."

Photography is all about producing an image by light exposure to get a good image, and using the appropriate lens to capture that image. Digital photography captures the image onto a sensor instead of a piece of photographic film. The digital picture is then transferred by the processor in your camera to a storage card. The principles of lighting, exposure, and depth of field remain the same as with analog (film) photography.

Basic Principles

The sensitivity of the card to light is determined by the ISO. The higher the ISO, the less light is required to get a good exposure, however the higher the ISO (asa) the grainier or more pixelated the image, so in dental photography we want to use the LOWEST

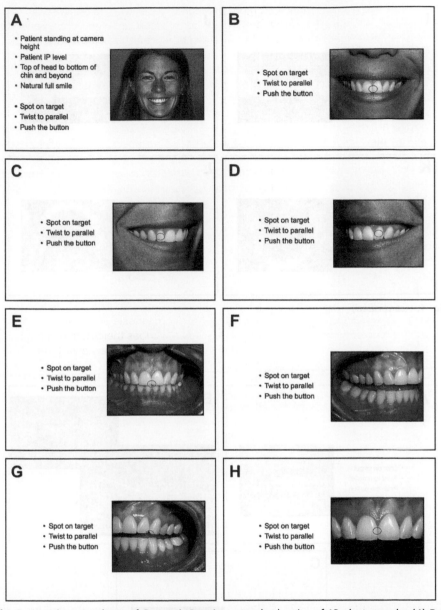

Fig. 1. American Academy of Cosmetic Dentistry standard series of 12 photographs. (*A*) Full face, (*B*) full smile, (*C*) right lateral smile, (*D*) left lateral smile, (*E*) anterior retracted closed, (*F*) right retracted, (*G*) left retracted, (*H*) 1:1 anterior retracted, (*I*) 1:1 right lateral, (*J*) 1:1 left lateral, (*K*) maxillary occlusal, and (*L*) mandibular occlusal.

ISO (asa) possible for that camera, usually 100 to 200 to have a clear, crisp, sharp photograph.

The amount of light that enters the camera is controlled by the aperture, the shutter speed, and the intensity of the light.

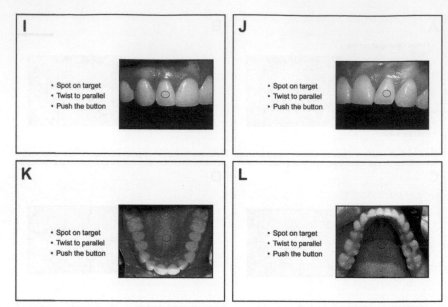

Fig. 1. (*continued*)

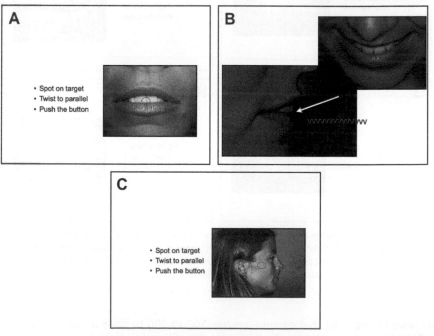

Fig. 2. Additional views for cosmetic dentistry. (*A*) Smile at rest, (*B*) IEP incisal edges touching vermillion border in "vvvvvv sounds" and IEP horizontal in "vvv" sounds, (*C*) right profile view.

Aperture and depth of field

The opening in the lens called the aperture. This aperture can be changed from large to small. A large opening lets a lot of light in, whereas a small opening lets only a little bit of light in; like opening your window blinds. The opening is measured as an f:stop. The larger opening has a smaller number, ie, f:2.8, whereas a small opening has a large number, ie, f:32. The size of the opening determines the depth of field. In close-up photography everything is magnified and the depth of field is magnified also.

It is important that in dental photography everything in the photograph must be in sharp focus (high depth of field), so we always need to use the highest aperture (f:stop) possible. This means we need to have as small an opening (aperture) in the lens as is possible (**Fig. 3**).

Shutter speed and sharpness

The next way to control the light is by the time we allow the light to enter the camera, the time the aperture stays open. This is controlled by the shutter. The longer the shutter stays open, the more light that enters, but the blurrier the photograph becomes because of camera shake and movement. A shutter speed of 1 second will allow 1 second's worth of light to enter the camera, whereas 1/125th of a second lets only a very small amount of light to enter the camera. Because in dental photography we will always be using a flash unit (strobe) to emit the light, and because the camera and the flash synchronize with each other at a specific shutter speed (designed by each camera), usually at 1/125th of a second, this no longer becomes a variable available to us and the shutter speed is predetermined as the flash synch shutter speed.

Lighting with flash (strobe)

The final method is to control the intensity of the light and that is controlled by the flash unit. In regular photography the flash unit is mounted on top of the camera. In dental photography this will cast a shadow into the mouth so the flash must be mounted on the end of the lens. The flash unit can be a ring light or a point source (either will work but the ring light is easier to use). The flash should be set on its maximum intensity to allow us to use the smallest aperture (highest f:stop means highest depth of

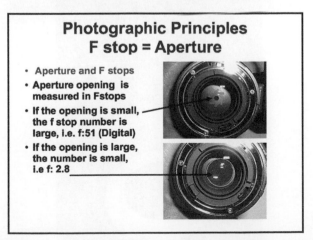

Fig. 3. Demonstrating aperture and depth of field. Open aperture, ie, f:4 gives limited depth of field where only the central part of the photograph is in focus. Small aperture, ie, f:32 gives maximum focus to all areas in the photograph.

field = maximum in focus). Remember when shopping for a ring light that some lights do not have the power to illuminate the inside of the mouth using a small aperture setting at ISO of 100 to 200 (**Fig. 4**).

The Lens

The most important piece of equipment is the lens. Macro photography is the ability to take close-up photographs. A true macro lens will give the practitioner the ability to "dial in" the magnification ratio required to take each type of photograph and get down to a 1:1 magnification ratio, which means the image in the camera is the same size as it is in real life! Watch out for the imitators here, there are lenses that are advertised as macro focus but they are not true macro lenses. Make sure the lens you purchase is a true 1:1 focusing macro lens.

A true macro lens will be able to give you a true rendition of the teeth without distortion. The focal length of the lens should be in the 90-mm to 105-mm range. The lens barrels can turn externally or internally. The external barrel will physically extend in and out. This allows you to place a piece of tape on the barrel and mark on the tape the magnification ratios, the exposure setting to help simplify the process of taking a perfect photo every time. The internal turning barrels will not extend in and out as the focusing is done internally. There will be a window in the lens to allow you to determine the magnification ratio desired (**Fig. 5**).

Magnification Ratio

Magnification ratio is predetermined by turning the lens barrel. In dental photography we use only 3 magnification ratios. The head shots are taken at 1:10 magnification; the smile views, occlusal views, and retracted views are taken using a 1:2 ratio; and the close-up shots are taken at a 1:1 magnification ratio. Simply turn the lens barrel and

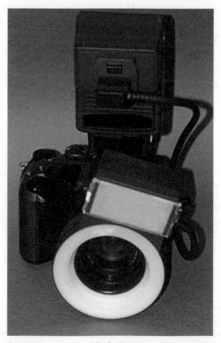

Fig. 4. Dental photography end-mounted lighting ring light, point light, combination.

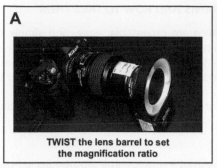
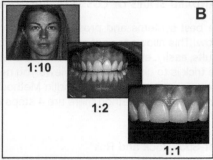

Fig. 5. (*A*) External barrel focusing macro lens with magnification ratios written on a sticker attached to the barrel for ease of use. (*B*) Magnification ratio views.

"dial in" the magnification ratio. This makes sure the view you take will be exactly the same every time.

The exposure will be the same for all the photos taken at each different magnification ratio. As you change the magnification ratio, you will then also need to change the f:stop (aperture) to correspond. This can be written down on the lens barrel itself for simplification.

Focusing

Usually when we take a photograph, we stand in one spot and push the autofocus, button which will automatically turn the lens barrel for us until the image comes into sharp focus. The problem is that this changes the magnification ratio.

In dental photography, the technique we use is a unique one. Maintaining the magnification ratio is of paramount importance, so we set the lens barrel to that magnification ratio by turning the lens barrel to that line, and instead of using the auto focus feature (turn off the auto focus feature), we focus by rocking back and forth until the image becomes clear! DO NOT TURN THE LENS BARREL TO FOCUS! (This is where a macro lens with an external barrel movement makes life easier so we can place tape on the barrel and simply turn to the correct magnification ratio.)

Camera Body

Any digital camera body that fits the lens you buy will do. The lens will be made to mount onto a particular camera, usually Nikon or Canon. Make sure the body matches the lens! Because we will be shooting everything in manual mode, we do not need to spend a lot on the camera body because we will not be using all the fancy automatic focusing features, the special automatic metering systems, and we do not even need the mega megapixels! A simple digital back that will allow you to shoot in manual mode with around 10 megapixels is more than sufficient!

SLR Versus Point and Shoot

There are varied opinions here. The costs of the systems are way down and the ease of use of the SLR system so far outweighs the point and shoot system's needed post picture manipulation and distortion that there is no question that the SLR option is the way to go. How many gadgets do you already have in your dental closet of shame that are unused because they are just too much of a hassle to use? Using photography in your practice will create an incredible return on investment. Do not skimp on the equipment that will get the job done quickly, easily, and predictably for you and your staff.

STANDARD SERIES OF COSMETIC PHOTOGRAPHS AND HOW TO TAKE THEM

The best systems and processes in the office are repeatable, easy, and simple to follow. This allows the entire dental team to be able to efficiently produce the desired results, easily, efficiently, and perfectly every time with a minimum of training required. The trick is to understand the views you need to take. Then you need to know how to take each view using the "Goodlin Method."

In the Goodlin Method there are 4 steps for every photograph: "Set-Spot-Rock and Roll."

"Set-Spot-Rock and Roll"

- Set the magnification ratio and the exposure f:stop number appropriate for that view.
- Position the focusing point onto the spot that is desired, eg, tip of nose, papilla.
- Rock forward and backward to "focus."
- Roll the camera like a steering wheel to make sure the image is straight.
- Push the button!

As an example, the procedure for the head shot would be as follows:

1. Turn the lens barrel to 1:10 magnification ratio. The aperture will be set to about f:4 (**Fig. 6**A).
2. Place the center focusing point on the spot. In this photo it is on the tip of the nose (see **Fig. 6**B).

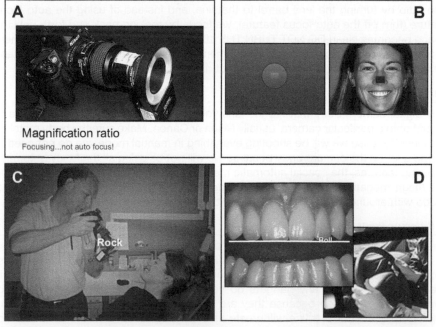

Fig. 6. (*A*) Set the magnification ratio. (*B*) Position the spot on the tip of the nose (full face view). (*C*) Rock back and forth to focus. (*D*) Roll to line up straight.

3. Rock your body forward and back slowly until the eyes look like they are clear and sharp (see **Fig. 6**C).
4. Now just roll the camera left and right like a steering wheel so that the picture is level now push the button (see **Fig. 6**D).

The Cosmetic Standard Series (17 views) is as follows:

1. Full Face 1:10
2. Right Profile view 1:10
3. Tooth show at rest 1:2 *Lick lips, swallow, slightly part your lips....Tooth show at rest is critical to determine IEP.*
4. Full exaggerated smile 1:2 EEEEEE
5. Horizontal view VVVVVV 1:2
6. Tipped forward VVVVVV 1:2
7. Right lateral smile view 1:2
8. Left lateral smile view 1:2
9. Retracted view anterior teeth closed 1:2
10. Retracted view anterior teeth slightly open 1:2
11. Right lateral retracted view 1:2 teeth closed 1:2
12. left lateral retracted view 1:2 teeth closed 1:2
13. Close-up anterior centrals view 1:1 with block-out paddle
14. Close-up right lateral retracted view 1:1 with block-out paddle
15. Close-up left lateral retracted view 1:1 with block-out paddle
16. Maxillary occlusal views 1:2 (photograph the reflection in an occlusal mirror)
17. Mandibular occlusal views 1:2 (photograph the reflection in an occlusal mirror) (**Figs. 7** and **8**).

DIAGNOSIS AND TREATMENT PLANNING
Anthropometrics and Cephalometrics

The concept of cephalometric measurements to determine orthodontic relationships between skeletal and dental patterns is not new to us. Anthropometric measurements[5]

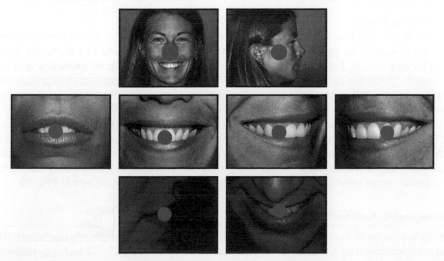

Fig. 7. Extraoral views with "focusing spot" marked.

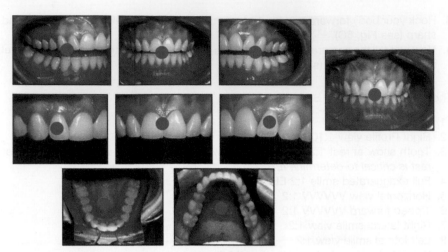

Fig. 8. Intraoral views with "focusing spot" marked.

are similarly used in cosmetic and plastic surgery all the time.[6] We in esthetic dentistry can use a combination of cephalometric and anthropometric principles to measure the dentofacial characteristics to assist in the diagnosis and treatment planning of the case, using the photographs we have taken during our diagnostic records appointment.

Facial proportion

A well proportioned face is divided into thirds, from forehead through the hairline, the eyebrows (Glabella), the base of the nose (Subnasion), and the edge of the chin (Menton). The proportional face is divided horizontally into fifths, edge of ear to outer canthis of eye, to ala of nose and repeated on the other side (**Fig. 9**).

We know that beauty is in the eye of the beholder, but the esthetic face has proportional relationships, dimensions, and contours and research has shown that these proportions are the same for most races, nationalities, and ethnic groups.

Golden proportion

The golden proportion has been around since before the building of the Parthenon in ancient Greece. The golden proportion is the key principle found in nature, art, and architecture and is the basis of the modern theory of dentofacial esthetics and is related to principles of cephalometrics and anthropometrics. Based on the principles of the ratio of 1.618: 1, this ratio is found to be the most pleasing for rectangles found in nature and transferred to manmade objects.[7]

The dento-facial characteristics we can determine from the golden proportion include width of both centrals to height of centrals, then by measuring height to width ratios, it has been determined that 78% is ideal.[8] The ratio of what the teeth should look like from a frontal view to get the proper dimensions of laterals and cuspids, and incisal edge position and vertical dimension of occlusion is shown in **Fig. 10**.

Photographic-Assisted Diagnosis

Using the Smile evaluation form, diagnostic parameters can be clearly correlated to the photographs that are taken in the standard cosmetic series.[9,10] This then enables the practitioner to diagnose the case using a set of photographs on which to make the

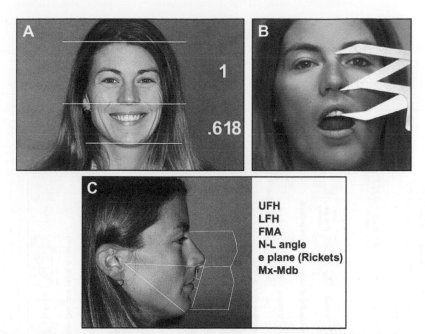

Fig. 9. (*A*) Proportions of the face extraorally. (*B*) Demonstration of the use of the golden proportion ruler to determine IEP. (*C*) Anthropometric measurements.

diagnostic analysis using the principles of cephalometrics, anthropometrics, and dentofacial esthetics.

TREATMENT PLANNING AND IMAGING

Once all of these factors have been determined, the clinician will be well on the way to a thorough and accurate diagnosis of the case and be able to create a comprehensive treatment plan for the patient. This can be achieved using computer programs designed to help the practitioner with the treatment planning process (GPS, Photoshop imaging) (**Fig. 11**). Once the preliminary treatment plan is created using photographic imaging, this can then be duplicated on a diagnostic wax-up model to be used to transfer the information to the mouth allowing the patient and practitioner to take the new smile for a test drive!

It is now simply a case of determining what goals we wish to achieve and what changes we want to make to the smile to maximize the esthetics and function.

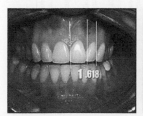 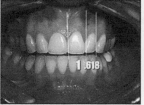 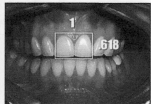

Fig. 10. Golden proportion ratios found intraorally.

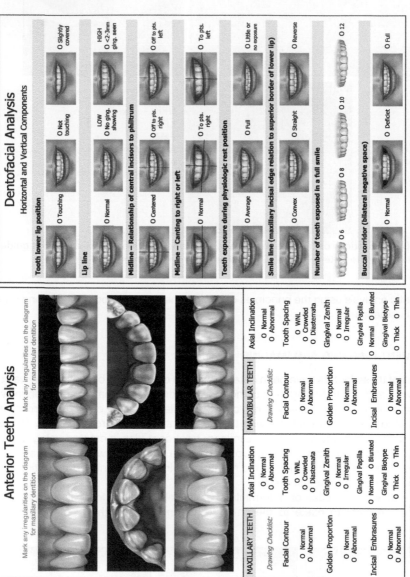

Fig. 11. (*A, B*) NYU Smile Design Evaluation Form.

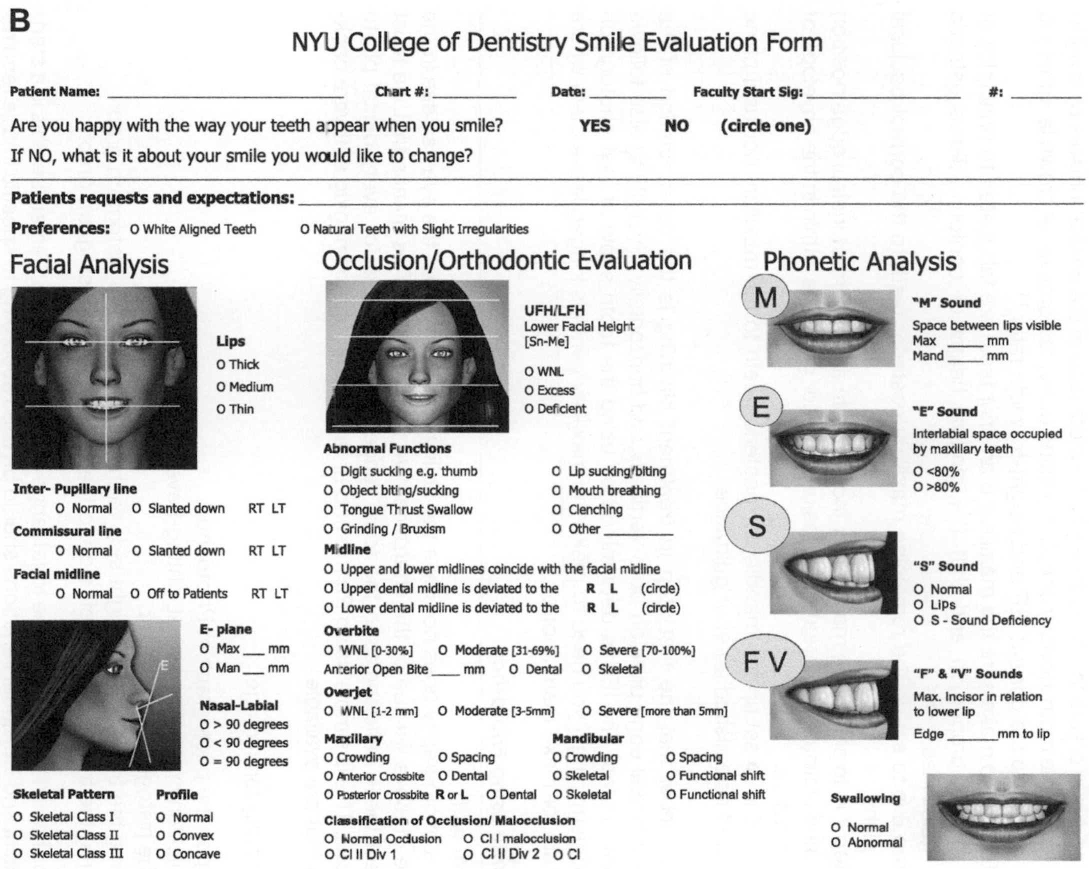

B

NYU College of Dentistry Smile Evaluation Form

Patient Name: _____   Chart #: _____   Date: _____   Faculty Start Sig: _____   #: _____

Are you happy with the way your teeth appear when you smile?   **YES   NO   (circle one)**

If NO, what is it about your smile you would like to change? _____

Patients requests and expectations:

Preferences: O White Aligned Teeth   O Natural Teeth with Slight Irregularities

Facial Analysis

Lips
- O Thick
- O Medium
- O Thin

Inter- Pupillary line
- O Normal   O Slanted down   RT   LT

Commissural line
- O Normal   O Slanted down   RT   LT

Facial midline
- O Normal   O Off to Patients   RT   LT

E- plane
- O Max ___ mm
- O Man ___ mm

Nasal-Labial
- O > 90 degrees
- O < 90 degrees
- O = 90 degrees

Skeletal Pattern
- O Skeletal Class I
- O Skeletal Class II
- O Skeletal Class III

Profile
- O Normal
- O Convex
- O Concave

Occlusion/Orthodontic Evaluation

UFH/LFH
Lower Facial Height [Sn-Me]
- O WNL
- O Excess
- O Deficient

Abnormal Functions
- O Digit sucking e.g. thumb
- O Object biting/sucking
- O Tongue Thrust Swallow
- O Grinding / Bruxism
- O Lip sucking/biting
- O Mouth breathing
- O Clenching
- O Other _____

Midline
- O Upper and lower midlines coincide with the facial midline
- O Upper dental midline is deviated to the   R   L   (circle)
- O Lower dental midline is deviated to the   R   L   (circle)

Overbite
- O WNL [0-30%]   O Moderate [31-69%]   O Severe [70-100%]
- Anterior Open Bite ___ mm   O Dental   O Skeletal

Overjet
- O WNL [1-2 mm]   O Moderate [3-5mm]   O Severe [more than 5mm]

Maxillary	Mandibular
O Crowding O Spacing	O Crowding O Spacing
O Anterior Crossbite O Dental	O Skeletal O Functional shift
O Posterior Crossbite R or L O Dental	O Skeletal O Functional shift

Classification of Occlusion/ Malocclusion
- O Normal Occlusion   O Cl I malocclusion
- O Cl II Div 1   O Cl II Div 2   O Cl

Phonetic Analysis

"M" Sound
Space between lips visible
Max ___ mm
Mand ___ mm

(M)

"E" Sound
Interlabial space occupied by maxillary teeth
- O <80%
- O >80%

(E)

"S" Sound
- O Normal
- O Lips
- O S - Sound Deficiency

(S)

"F" & "V" Sounds
Max. Incisor in relation to lower lip
Edge ___ mm to lip

(FV)

Swallowing
- O Normal
- O Abnormal

Fig. 11. (continued)

Treatment planning is very similar to the procedures we follow in setting up the full denture case.

Step 1 is to determine the correct occlusion rim height (incisal edge position vertically and horizontally and maxillary occlusal plane).

Step 2 is to create the midline position.

Step 3 is to create maxillary incisor inclination to stay within the neutral zone.

Step 4 is to create the correct height-to-width ratio of the central incisors by lengthening the tooth incisally or apically using ortho, restorative, or crown lengthening to create the correct IEP and height-to-width ratio.[11]

Step 5 is to make sure the maxillary 6 anterior teeth are fabricated to principles of golden proportion and that the gingival height of contour follows esthetic guidelines.[12,13]

Step 6 is to set up the remaining maxillary posterior teeth to the correct occlusal plane.

Step 7 is to set up the mandibular incisor teeth at the correct incisal edge position and inclination to create the desired anterior guidance within in the envelope of function.

Step 8 is to set up the mandibular posterior teeth to the maxillary occlusal plane and established anterior guidance.

Remember that the first step in treatment planning is the determination of the correct incisal edge position both vertically and horizontally. Everything else follows this initial step. The IEP is determined by using the tooth show at rest photograph and determining if you need to make the maxillary centrals longer, leave them where they are, or make them shorter.

Imaging using Photoshop

Global edits

Digital photography does not have the ability to recreate what the eye can see in the range of tones we see or the sharpness we percieve.[14–18] This means that we must correct these deficiencies in the tonal range and sharpness for every digital photo we take. This is simple using Photoshop or many other photo imaging software packages that are available.

Correcting tonal range:

1. Open the photograph in Photoshop
2. Click on Image-Enhance-Lighting-Levels
3. The histogram will appear
4. Drag the triangle on the right side to the right side of the histogram graph
5. Drag the triangle on the left side to the left side of the histogram graph.

You have now corrected the tonal range of the photograph. Remember this is a starting point and individual variations should be used according to specific image requirements (**Fig. 12**).

Correcting sharpness:

1. The photo is already open in Photoshop
2. Click Filter-Sharpen-Unsharp mask
3. Amount = 100% Threshold = 0

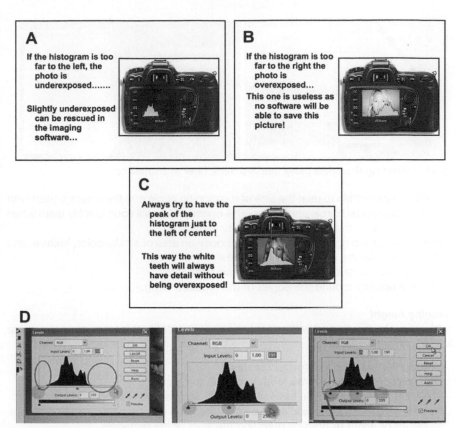

Fig. 12. Correcting tonal range using histograms: (*A*) too dark, (*B*) too light, (*C*) correct position of histogram, (*D*) global edit correction of tonal range.

4. Set the radius according to the magnification ratio:
    1:10 = 1.0
    1:2 = 3.0
    1:1 = 5.0

5. Click OK.

Remember this is a starting point and individual variations should be used according to specific image requirements (**Fig. 13**).

Imaging is used to help the practitioner see what treatment should be provided the patient as well as showing the patient to help him or her understand the process and importance of cosmetic dentistry. The photos can then be easily dragged and dropped into a quick PowerPoint (keynote - Mac) presentation or simply use your iPad or laptop computer to show the patient chairside. It is very easy using the basic Photoshop tools and after a few times of practicing your skills it will be quick and simple to show your patients their imaged smile. This is one of the best marketing/sales tools you will ever use!

Image old fillings with clone tool
This tool will pick up a small part of a photo and place it over top of another area.

Click on clone tool.

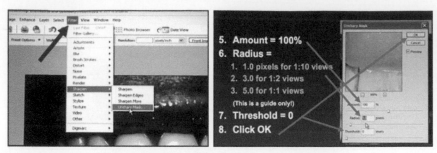

Fig. 13. Correcting sharpness using unsharp mask filter in Photoshop.

There are 2 controls to use: the size of the cloning circle and the opacity. Start with a medium-sized circle and about 50% opacity. You will soon quickly learn when to use 100% and when to use opacity variations.

Press CMND and right click to pick up (choose an area of similar color, texture, and exposure as the area you want to hide).

Place cursor circle over area to clone and right click.

Vary the opacity around the edges of the repaired filling.

Changing height

Width ratios, ie, length and width of teeth (this is a great tool for imaging a diastema closure).

Choose the marquis tool (rectangle dash).

Drag and drop to outline the tooth you want to change.

Press Ctl C then Ctl V (you have now cloned and pasted the tooth onto itself.

Now press Ctl T. The rectangle will be activated and you will now be able to change height or width or both by dragging the lines of the rectangle.

Once you have the shape you want, press enter.

Now use the eraser tool to smooth out the corners and embrasure spaces.

Tooth whitening

Quick selection tool and select the teeth in the smile.

Fine tune your selection using the lasso tool + and −.

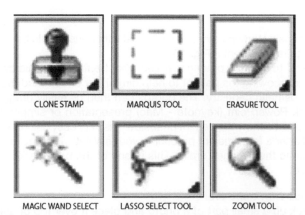

Fig. 14. Photoshop tool icons: Clone, Marquis, Erasure, Magic Wand Select, Lasso Select, Zoom.

Once you have the selection you wish to work with (outlined with "marching ants"), press Image-Adjust-lighting-brightness/contrast…. move the brightness slider over until the teeth are the brightness you desire to simulate whitening.

You can also use Lighting-levels or Lighting-exposure or color-adjust hue/saturation and adjust the sliders for decrease saturation and increase brightness to accomplish the same thing.

Using these 6 basic tools will give you a great start in being able to image your patient photographs and show the patient what they could look like following cosmetic dental procedures (**Fig. 14**).

REFERENCES

1. Wikipedia. "Standard of Practice."
2. Goodlin RM. The standard series of intra oral photographs. Univ Tor Dent J 1979; 14(3):4–10.
3. Spear F. Making good images perfect DVD collection. Seattle (WA): Spear Institute; 2008.
4. Goodlin R. The complete guide to dental photography. Montreal (Canada): Michael Publishing; 1987.
5. Ward RE. Facial morphology as determined by anthropometry: keeping it simple. J Craniofac Genet Dev Biol 1989;9:45–60.
6. Rogers BO. The role of physical anthropology in plastic surgery. Clin Plast Surg 1974;1:434–98.
7. Rickets RM. The golden divider. J Clin Orthod 1981;15:752–9.
8. Levin EI. Dental esthetics and golden proportion. J Prosthet Dent 1978;40: 244–52.
9. Goodlin R. Photographic assisted diagnosis. Cdn J Cos Dent 2005;1(1):6–12.
10. Calamia J, Levine JB, Lipp MJ. NYU College of Dentistry Smile Evaluation Form. In: "A multidisciplinary approach to the indirect esthetic treatment of diastemata" functional esthetics and restorative dentistry dentalaegis. Series 1, issue 3, 2007.
11. Goodlin R. Gingival aesthetics. J Oral Health 2003;5:247–51.
12. Rickets RE. The biological significance of the divine proportion. Am J Orthop 1982;81:351–70.
13. Blitz N, Steel C, Whilhite C. Diagnosis and treatment evaluation in cosmetic dentistry. Madison (WI): AACD; 2002.
14. Goodlin R. Photographic imaging using Photoshop. 2009. Available at: www.smiledental.ca. Interactive DVD.
15. Cunningham M. Measuring the physical in attractiveness. J Pers Soc Psychol 1986;50:925–35.
16. Preston J. The golden proportion revisited. J Esthet Dent 1993;5:247–51.
17. Rickets RE. The divine proportion in facial aesthetics. Clin Plast Surg 1982;9: 401–22.
18. Woodside DG. Cephalometric roentgenography. In: James W, editor. Clinical dentistry, Clark. Toronto (Canada): Harper and Row; 1976.

Whitening the Single Discolored Tooth

So Ran Kwon, DDS, MS, PhD

KEYWORDS

- Single discolored tooth • Traumatic injury
- Bleaching techniques • Complications

The single discolored tooth can be a challenge in obtaining an esthetic outcome in the anterior region (**Figs. 1–3**). Treatment options can vary from restorative procedures such as crowns, veneers, or bonding to more conservative bleaching treatments. The long-term success of the treatment is dictated by proper diagnosis and treatment planning. The cause and severity of the discoloration has to be carefully evaluated when planning for bleaching options. The vitality of the pulp, presence and absence of symptoms, and periapical pathoses usually determine whether an external or internal bleaching approach will be considered.

THE INITIAL EXAMINATION

Patients presenting with a single discolored tooth should always be questioned about any history of traumatic injury to the tooth. Regardless of the status of the pulp, a former trauma might have caused bleeding into the dentinal tubules resulting in a dark brown to black discoloration. The baseline color may be evaluated with the VITA Classical shade guide (VITA, Bad Sackingen, Germany) or the VITA Bleached-guide (VITA, Bad Sackingen, Germany). However, single discolored teeth usually are outside the range of commercial shade guides so that technology-based color measuring devices such as the VITA Easyshade Compact (VITA, Bad Sackingen, Germany), Spectroshade Micro (MHT, Verona, Italy), or CrystalEye (Olympus, Tokyo, Japan) may be used to obtain a more objective evaluation of the tooth color at baseline and accurate data on the color change before and after bleaching. Another important consideration when evaluating baseline tooth color is the color of the root and the thickness and level of the gingiva. The dentin in the root is different from the anatomic crown, and does not bleach well if at all, regardless of whether internal or external bleaching is attempted.[1] Radiographs, vitality testing with ice and electric pulp testing, and transillumination are additional procedures that should be performed to assess whether root canal treatment is indicated prior to bleaching (**Figs. 4–6**).

The case included in this article has been presented at the 2nd Annual Meeting of the Society of Color and Appearance in Dentistry, September 24, 2010.
Department of Operative Dentistry, College of Dentistry, University of Iowa, Iowa City, IA 52242-1001, USA
E-mail address: soran-kwon@uiowa.edu

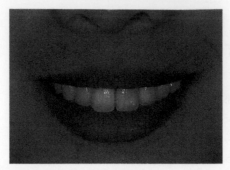

Fig. 1. Preoperative view of full smile of the patient.

If the tooth is nonvital and there is absence of periapical radiolucency and symptoms, endodontic treatment is usually not recommended. However, if the pulp canal is severely obliterated, performing endodontic treatment before the development of a periapical radiolucency may prevent difficulty and complications associated with these teeth, and also increase the success rate for teeth treated without periapical radiolucencies versus teeth treated with periapical radiolucencies.[2]

CAUSES OF DISCOLORATION

The tooth can discolor from extravasations of blood components into the dentinal tubules associated with pulp extirpation or traumatic injury.[3] The blood cells undergo hemolysis and release iron, which reacts with hydrogen sulfide, a metabolic by-product of bacteria, to form iron sulfide, which causes the gray staining of the tooth.[4] Incomplete removal of pulpal debris, especially in the pulp horn area, is another cause of discoloration in a single root-filled tooth.[5] Root-filling materials can also cause coronal discoloration.[6] Bleaching can be effective in removing stains depending on the substance. However, discoloration caused by metallic ions cannot be removed by whitening treatments.[7] If the pulp survives a traumatic injury, it can undergo pulp canal obliteration, also referred to as calcific metamorphosis. Calcific metamorphosis is characterized by rapid deposition of hard tissue beginning within the pulp chamber and continuing along the root canal space, resulting in a yellow to brown discoloration of the clinical crown. Studies indicate that 1% to 16% of calcific metamorphosis cases will eventually undergo pulp necrosis, so that it is advisable to manage cases demonstrating calcific metamorphosis through observation and periodic examination.[8]

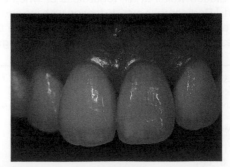

Fig. 2. Frontal view of discolored left central incisor.

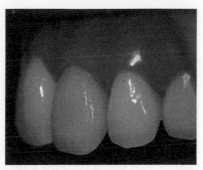

Fig. 3. Lateral view of discolored left central incisor.

BLEACHING MATERIALS FOR THE SINGLE DISCOLORED TOOTH

Bleaching of discolored teeth was first attempted on nonvital teeth with the use of various bleaching materials including chlorinated lime, oxalic acid, sodium peroxide, sodium hypochlorite, and mixtures of 25% hydrogen peroxide in 75% ether (pyrozone).[9] Hydrogen peroxide, the most commonly used bleaching material nowadays, was reported by Harlan in 1885.[10] Hydrogen peroxide was placed into the pulp cavity at chair-side and replaced periodically or activated with electric current,[11] heat,

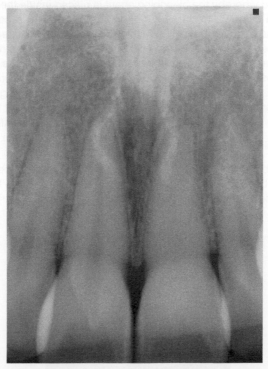

Fig. 4. Periapical radiograph. Note the pulp canal obliteration state on the left central incisor.

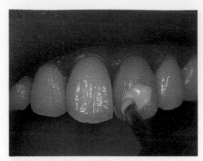

Fig. 5. Vitality testing with electric pulp testing exhibited a positive response.

or light[12–15] to speed up the bleaching process. The acceleration was assumed to follow the Q_{10} rule that for every 10°C increase in temperature, the reaction rate increases 2 times. The use of a mixture of sodium perborate and distilled water was described by Salvas[16] and reconsidered by Spasser[17] as the walking bleach technique. This technique is still widely accepted, with various modifications in the bleaching agent placed in the chamber. Nutting and Poe[18] used a mixture of sodium perborate and 30% hydrogen peroxide to speed up the process. Since the first publication on night guard bleaching with the use of 10% carbamide peroxide,[19] mixtures of sodium perborate and carbamide peroxide of different concentrations have been proposed.[20,21] The use of carbamide peroxide in nonvital bleaching has also changed the delivery method whereby the bleaching agent is placed inside the chamber as well as the outside in a custom-fitted tray.[22–24] The use of carbamide peroxide has been advocated because of its neutral pH and slow release of active ingredients. However, when 30% hydrogen peroxide is mixed with sodium perborate in a ratio of 2:1 (g/mL) the pH of the mixture is alkaline, which favors the effectiveness of the bleaching agent. So far there seems to be no agreement on which bleaching material is best, but it seems prudent to understand the chemistry of each bleaching agent and apply it cautiously to the proposed treatment technique.

BLEACHING TECHNIQUES

There are several bleaching techniques available for the single discolored tooth. The decision is mainly based on the vitality of the tooth and whether the treatment should be performed in the office or at home, or a combination of both.

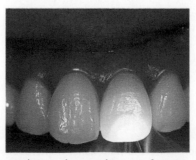

Fig. 6. Transillumination is used to evaluate existence of severe crack lines.

Single-Tooth In-Office Bleaching

A single discolored tooth without any symptoms, no periapical pathosis, and a questionable response to vitality testing is a good candidate for in-office bleaching with highly concentrated hydrogen peroxide that is commonly used in power bleaching for vital teeth.

Treatment Sequence
- Evaluate the color with a shade guide or a color measurement device (**Figs. 7** and **8**).
- Clean the tooth with a slurry of pumice and rubber-cup.
- Isolate the tooth on the facial and lingual side with a resin barrier or rubber dam (**Fig. 9**).
- Apply highly concentrated bleaching agent on the facial and lingual.
- Place a precut linear low-density polyethylene wrap onto the bleaching agent to prevent evaporation of the bleaching agent and inadvertent contact with the patient's soft tissue (**Fig. 10**).[25]
- Activate the bleaching agent with light (optional).
- Remove bleaching agent after 40 to 60 minutes with a high suction tip or a small cotton pellet.
- Rinse and remove the resin barrier or rubber dam.
- Evaluate the tooth color and reappoint patient for several in-office bleaching sessions until the desired shade is obtained.

Single-Tooth Tray Bleaching

The indication for single-tooth tray bleaching is similar to single-tooth in-office bleaching. However, if the patient shows good cooperation and prefers to perform the treatment at home, tray bleaching is highly recommended.

Treatment Sequence
- Take an alginate impression of the whole arch.
- Pour the impression with plaster and avoid any bubbles or defects.
- Trim the cast so that the occlusal surface is parallel to the base (**Fig. 11**).
- Use an Omnivacuum machine to fabricate a custom-fitted tray.

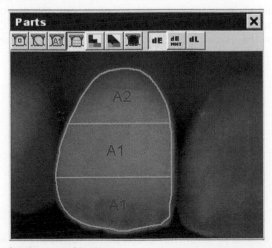

Fig. 7. Color map of right central incisor.

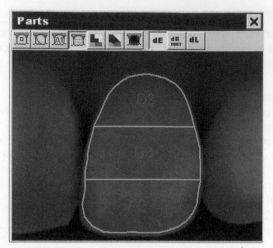

Fig. 8. Color map of discolored left central incisor.

- Trim the tray in a straight pattern on the facial and lingual side.
- Mark the tooth to be bleached and scallop the facial and lingual side of the tray, only at the marked tooth area (**Fig. 12**).
- Disinfect the tray with a cleaning solution in an ultrasonic cleaner.
- Deliver the tray and home bleaching gel (10%–20% carbamide peroxide gel).
- Instruct the patient to place the bleaching gel only at the discolored tooth and wear the tray overnight.
- Reappoint the patient to evaluate the progress of the treatment.
- Evaluate the color of the tooth and the bleaching change relevant to the adjacent teeth (**Figs. 13–15**).

Thermocatalytic Bleaching

The thermocatalytic bleaching technique is one of the oldest forms of bleaching nonvital teeth in the office. However, the use of highly concentrated hydrogen peroxide in a liquid state requires utmost attention, and the use of heat has often been associated with the development of cervical root resorption. Consequently the performance of the thermocatalytic bleaching technique is decreasing.

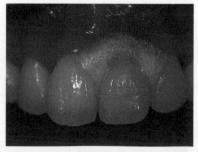

Fig. 9. Isolation of discolored tooth with a resin barrier (OpalDam, Ultradent Products Inc, South Jordan, UT, USA).

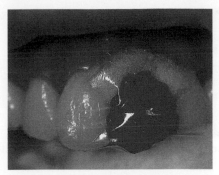

Fig. 10. Placement of a 38% hydrogen peroxide gel (Opalescence Boost, Ultradent Product Inc, South Jordan, UT, USA) and a linear low-density polyethylene wrap.

Walking Bleach Technique

The use of an intracoronal filling of sodium perborate combined with water or hydrogen peroxide continues until today, and has been shown to be a successful treatment for bleaching nonvital teeth.[26]

Treatment Sequence
- Evaluate the existing root canal filling on the radiograph.
- Isolate the tooth with a well-fitting rubber dam.
- Clean the pulp chamber and the pulp horns of any debris or pulpal remnants.
- Remove the gutta percha root canal filling material with a heated instrument or a low-speed small round burr to 2 mm below the cementoenamel junction.
- Place a cervical barrier of 2 mm thickness with glass-ionomer cement or flowable resin to prevent the leakage of hydrogen peroxide into the surrounding alveolar bone.
- Mix sodium perborate with water or hydrogen peroxide in a ratio of 2:1 (g/mL) to a thick mix.
- Place the mixture into the pulp chamber with an amalgam carrier or an applicator.
- Use a damp cotton pellet to remove excess material to allow space for the temporary filling material.
- Use Cavit or glass-ionomer cement as a temporary filling material to properly seal the access cavity.

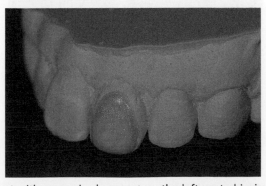

Fig. 11. Trimmed cast with reservoir placement on the left central incisor.

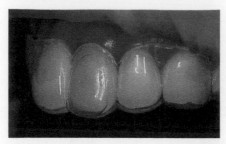

Fig. 12. The custom fitted tray is scalloped only on the single discolored tooth.

- Recall the patient after 3 to 5 days to evaluate the progress of the treatment, and repeat the walking bleach procedure 3 to 5 times until the color matches that of the adjacent teeth.
- The final composite restoration should be placed 2 to 3 weeks after the last walking bleach procedure to allow for the color to stabilize, and to allow for the recovery of bond strength to tooth structure that is usually compromised immediately after bleaching.[27]

Inside-Outside Closed Bleaching

This technique comprises the combination of walking bleach and the single-tooth tray bleaching to speed up the bleaching process and to reduce multiple appointments in the office.

Inside-Outside Open Bleaching

The inside-outside open bleaching technique is indicated in patients with good cooperation, because the bleaching agent has to be applied outside and inside within the pulp chamber.

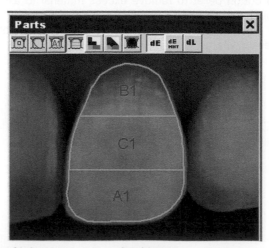

Fig. 13. Color map of left central incisor after bleaching.

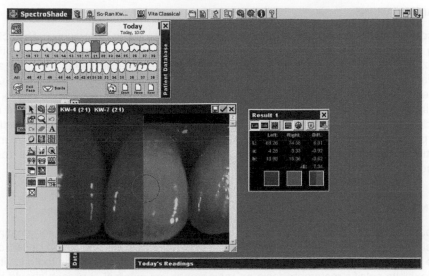

Fig. 14. Split-tooth image showing the difference of color change before and after bleaching, ΔE = 7.34.

Treatment Sequence

- Take an alginate impression of the whole arch and fabricate a custom-fitted tray as for a single-tooth tray bleaching.
- Evaluate the existing root canal filling and place a cervical barrier of 2 mm thickness.
- Instruct the patient to fill the custom-fitted tray of the marked tooth on the labial side and also fill the pulp chamber with 10% to 20% carbamide peroxide. The tray can be worn every day, overnight until the color of the discolored tooth matches that of adjacent teeth.
- Show the patient how to irrigate the open chamber when debris has accumulated inside the chamber.
- Place the final composite restoration 2 to 3 weeks after the last bleaching gel application.

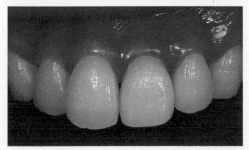

Fig. 15. Natural blend-in of color with adjacent teeth after combined in-office and single-tooth tray bleaching.

COMPLICATIONS

Occurrence of external cervical root resorption has been linked to intracoronal bleaching using hydrogen peroxide. The exact mechanism is still unknown, but it is hypothesized that hydrogen peroxide penetrates into the alveolar bone, causing an inflammatory response.[28] It has also been postulated that hydrogen peroxide denatures the collagen initiating a foreign body reaction,[29] or decreases the pH resulting in increased osteoclastic activity.[30] All theories are based on the microleakage of hydrogen peroxide into the surrounding alveolar bone. Therefore it seems essential to place a barrier in order to seal the patent dentinal tubules, especially in young patients with wide open tubules, to prevent the development of cervical root resorption.

SUMMARY

Bleaching is the most conservative, economical, and safe approach for treating a single discolored tooth. The bleaching technique employed should be based on the vitality of the tooth and the cooperation of the patient. Whenever the tooth is vital or exhibits calcific metamorphosis on radiographs, an external approach should be used. In a nonvital tooth with existing root canal fillings, the chamber can be used for the walking bleach technique or for the inside-outside bleaching technique. Caution should be exercised as to the time of the placement of the final composite resin restoration in the pulp chamber. Bonding to the enamel and dentin is affected immediately after bleaching, so that the final restoration should be placed 2 to 3 weeks after the last bleaching session. Failure to do so might affect the long-term color stability of the treated tooth.

REFERENCES

1. Haywood VB, Diangelis AJ. Bleaching the single dark tooth. Inside Dent 2010; 6(September):42–52.
2. daCunho FM, deSouza IM, Monnerat J. Pulp canal obliteration subsequent to trauma: perforation management with MTA followed by canal localization and obturation. Brazilian J Dent Traumatology 2009;1(2):64–8.
3. Goldstein RE, Garber DA. Complete dental bleaching. Berlin: Quintessence; 1995.
4. Grossmann LI. Endodontic practice. 5th edition. Philadelphia: Lea and Febiger; 1960.
5. Brown G. Factors influencing successful bleaching of the discolored root-filled tooth. Oral Surg Oral Med Oral Pathol 1965;20:238–44.
6. Van der Burgt TP, Plaesschaert AJ. Tooth discoloration induced by dental materials. Oral Surg Oral Med Oral Pathol 1985;60:666–9.
7. Glockner K, Ebeleseder K. Indikationen und Grenzfaelle fuer das Bleichen von devitalen verfaerbten Frontzaehnen. Quintessenz 1993;44:519–27 [in German].
8. Amir FA, Gutmann JL, Witherspoon DE. Calcific metamorphosis: a challenge in endodontic diagnosis and treatment. Quintessence Int 2001;32:447–55.
9. Attin T, Paque F, Ajam F, et al. Review of the current status of tooth whitening with the walking bleach technique. Int Endod J 2003;36:313–29.
10. Harlan AW. The removal of stains from teeth caused by administration of medical agents and the bleaching of a pulpless tooth. Am J Dent Sci 1884/1885;18:521.
11. Westlake A. Bleaching teeth by electricity. Am J Dent Sci 1895;29:101.

12. Rosenthal P. The combined use of ultra-violet rays and hydrogen dioxide for bleaching teeth. Dent Cosmos 1911;53:246–7.
13. Prinz H. Recent improvements in tooth bleaching. A clinical syllabus. Dent Cosmos 1924;66:558–60.
14. Brininstool CL. Vapor bleaching. Dent Cosmos 1913;55:532.
15. Merrel JH. Bleaching of discolored pulpless tooth. J Can Dent Assoc 1954;20:380.
16. Salvas CJ. Perborate as a bleaching agent. J Am Dent Assoc 1938;25:324.
17. Spasser HF. A simple bleaching technique using sodium perborate. N Y State Dent J 1961;27:332–4.
18. Nutting EB, Poe GS. A new combination for bleaching teeth. J South Calif Dent Assoc 1963;31:289.
19. Haywood VB, Heymann HO. Nightguard vital bleaching. Quintessence Int 1989;20:173–6.
20. Aldecoa EA, Mayordomo FG. Modified internal bleaching of severe tetracycline discolorations: a 6-year clinical evaluation. Quintessence Int 1992;23:83–9.
21. Yui KC, Rodrigues JR, Mancini MN, et al. Ex vivo evaluation of the effectiveness of bleaching agents on the shade alteration of blood-stained teeth. Int Endod J 2008;41:485–92.
22. Liebenberg WH. Intracoronal lightening of discolored pulpless teeth: a modified walking bleach technique. Quintessence Int 1997;28:771–7.
23. Settembrini L, Gultz J, Kaim J, et al. A technique for bleaching non-vital teeth: inside/outside bleaching. J Am Dent Assoc 1997;128:1283 4.
24. Carillo A, Trevino MV, Haywood VB. Simultaneous bleaching of vital and an open chamber non-vital tooth with 10% carbamide peroxide. Quintessence Int 1998;29:643–8.
25. Kwon SR, Ko SH, Greenwall L. Tooth whitening in esthetic dentistry. Berlin: Quintessence; 2009.
26. Attin T, Kielbassa AM. Die Bleichbehandlung-ein fester Bestandteil aesthetischer Zahnheilkunde. Zahnärztl Mitt 1995;85:2674–80 [in German].
27. Shinohara MS, Rodrigues A, Pimenta AF. In vitro microleakage of composite restorations after non-vital bleaching. Quintessence Int 2001;32:413–7.
28. Harrington GW, Natkin E. External resorption associated with bleaching of pulpless teeth. J Endod 1979;5:344–8.
29. Lado EA, Stanley HR, Weismann MI. Cervical root resorption in bleached teeth. Oral Surg Oral Med Oral Pathol 1983;55:78–80.
30. McCormick JE, Weine FS, Maggio JD. Tissue pH of developing periapical lesions in dogs. J Endod 1983;9:47–51.

In-office Vital Bleaching with Adjunct Light

Joe C. Ontiveros, DDS, MS

KEYWORDS

- Tooth bleaching • Tooth whitening • Bleaching light
- Whitening lamp • Tooth color • Dental shade guide
- Power bleaching • In-office bleaching

E.P. Wright, the nineteenth-century dental researcher and scholar, stated that "there is no higher glory for one who professes the healing art [of dentistry] than of preserving the natural tissues." He published a paper in 1890 entitled "bleaching of discolored dentin practically considered."[1] His sentiment still rings true and this is why nearly 120 years after his publication the conservative nature of the in-office bleaching procedure still appeals to both patients and dentists alike. However, unlike those early years of bleaching when the procedure was preserved for severe discoloration, usually a single tooth caused by the loss of vitality, it is now common to perform complete dental bleaching on vital teeth. Vital bleaching was introduced to the profession in 1989, using 10% carbamide peroxide in a custom bleaching tray for at-home use.[2] The dental bleaching procedure was no longer reserved for the single discolored tooth, but multiple vital teeth could be whitened for cosmetic reasons as patients presented with mild to moderate stains on all the teeth.

Although home-based whitening methods and materials have a prominent place in the dental market,[3] in-office bleaching for vital teeth, especially with the use of adjunct light, has seen a steady increase in popularity in the last decade. The use of light as an adjunct to whitening has most likely seen its demand increase because of the extensive marketing that has occurred and the visibility of the procedure outside the dental office. For instance, whitening with supplemental lighting appears on television reality shows, billboards, and at kiosks in shopping malls.

Light-assisted, in-office bleaching methods use higher concentrations of peroxide in conjunction with supplemental light to enhance the effect of tooth whitening. These methods tend to appeal to patients who have a desire for rapid results and perhaps those not interested in wearing custom trays at night or those not successful with over-the-counter products. Dentists must be informed about the advantages and

The author has nothing to disclose.

The University of Texas Health Science Center at Houston Dental Branch, Department of Restorative and Biomaterials, 6516 MD Anderson Boulevard, Suite 480, Houston, TX 77030, USA

E-mail address: joe.c.ontiveros@uth.tmc.edu

doi:10.1016/j.cden.2011.01.002
dental.theclinics.com

disadvantage of these methods and be able to make decisions for offering in-office bleaching with adjunct light based on sound evidence and well-controlled scientific studies.

PROFESSIONAL SUPERVISION: DIAGNOSIS AND REGULATION

Important issues surrounding the use of whitening lamps to bleach teeth revolve around the concern for the health and safety of the patient. The appearance of tooth-whitening kiosks in malls, salons, and other nondental settings has caused some states to take action in banning nondental businesses. Although the employees of these businesses may wear white coats or scrubs and call themselves teeth-whitening professionals or cosmetic teeth-whitening specialists, they typically have no dental education. Proponents of light-assisted whitening outside the dental office may claim their services fall within the definition for cosmetic of the US Food and Drug Administration (FDA). However, states such as Alabama for example have been successful at making the case that these businesses are practicing dentistry without a license.[4]

The cases against nondental providers are not directly against the administration of bleaching agents because the employees typically have the patients insert the product in their own mouths, but against a lack of training in matters such as treatment planning, sterilization, infection control, pain management, and emergency procedures, including the management of allergic reactions. In late 2009, the American Dental Association petitioned the FDA to establish appropriate classifications for tooth-whitening chemicals.[5] Until the laws are clarified, state dental boards continue to work through their legislatures to ensure the health and safety of the people who resort to tooth-whitening services provided in nondental settings.

In the dental office, tooth whitening begins with a proper examination to screen for the presence of any dental disease. In addition to radiographs to rule out endodontic disease or decay, a treatment plan must be formulated to manage existing restorations, and the cause of the discoloration must be determined to initiate an effective bleaching strategy.

CASE SELECTION/MINIMIZING RISKS AND SIDE EFFECTS

A through clinical examination should reveal not only cases that are suitable for in-office bleaching with adjunct light, such as teeth with mild to moderate discoloration (**Fig. 1**), but also teeth that are not suitable using this method, such as the single discolored tooth (**Fig. 2**A) or the patient who presents with teeth beyond the shade of the lightest tab on a standard shade guide (see **Fig. 2**B). The patient who presents with severe intrinsic staining (see **Fig. 2**C) may also be better served with long-term at-home bleaching.

Greater tooth sensitivity has been reported with in-office bleaching with adjunct light compared with no light.[6] Risk factors for sensitivity, such as existing decay, gingival recession, cervical abrasions, or a history of sensitivity, should be identified during the review of the patient's dental history. Patient identified with existing tooth sensitivity may prebrush for about 2 weeks with a toothpaste containing potassium nitrate to help minimize sensitivity.[7,8] Patients can also be provided with 600 mg of ibuprofen 30 minutes before the in-office procedure to help reduce sensitivity. However, a recent study showed that patients who received ibuprofen 30 minutes before an appointment compared with patients who received a placebo capsule reported the same level of sensitivity 1 hour after the in-office procedure, which continued up to 24 hours.[9] This finding means that additional doses of ibuprofen may be necessary after the

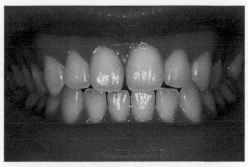

Fig. 1. Patients with mild to moderate yellow extrinsically discolored teeth may be good candidates for in-office bleaching with adjunct light.

in-office bleaching procedure to prevent postoperative sensitivity. Applying 4% to 6% potassium nitrate gel on the lingual surface of the teeth during the appointment is another strategy to minimize tooth sensitivity.

Concentrations of hydrogen peroxide between 15% and 40% are used for professional in-office bleaching, which poses a risk of chemical tissue damage. Also the human eyes and oral soft tissue should be protected from the blue light or ultraviolet (UV) radiation emitted from the bleaching light. A recent study reported the health risk from optical radiation of 7 commercially available bleaching lamps.[10] This study reported that most of the lamps exceeded the standards set for exposure limits for direct blue light to patients' eyes before the recommended treatment times had elapsed. One light even exceeded the exposure limits set for reflected blue light within the recommended treatment time. Although the potential health risk for emission of blue light and UV hazard were all classified as low to moderate-low risk according to safety standards, these findings highlight the importance of proper barriers on all exposed tissues (**Fig. 3**A). Also to minimize reflective radiation, protective light guides surrounding the end of the light source are recommended (see **Fig. 3**B), and protective eyewear for patients is essential (see **Fig. 3**C).

SETTING EXPECTATIONS OF TREATMENT TIME

When reviewing treatment options and setting expectations with patients regarding bleaching vital teeth, we must first discuss the advantages and disadvantages of in-office versus at-home techniques. The primary advantage most sought after from

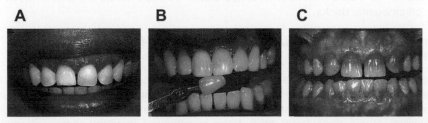

Fig. 2. Three cases that may not be best suited for bleaching with adjunct light. (*A*) A patient who presents with a single discolored tooth. (*B*) A patient who already presents with extremely light teeth. (*C*) A patient who presents with intrinsic staining caused by tetracycline.

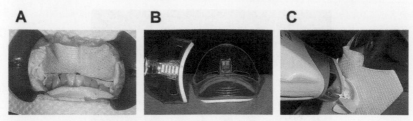

Fig. 3. Proper protection from scatter and direct radiant energy is essential for the in-office bleaching procedure with adjunct light. (*A*) All soft tissues are protected with a resin barrier and multiple 2 × 2 gauze. Only the lower arch is isolated in this image for research purposes. (*B*) A protective light guide that connects to the face of the lamp head is used to minimize indirect scattered radiation. (*C*) Light-protective glasses are provided to the patient during treatment.

patients attracted to in-office bleaching is the expectation of rapid results. The question of how much time is saved with in-office techniques is not easy to answer, because results can vary among patients and depend on the cause of the stains, but some general expectation should be discussed based on available clinical evidence. Seven days of at-home bleaching with 10% carbamide has been shown to be equivalent to 3 15-minute applications of 38% hydrogen peroxide[11] or 5 days of at-home bleach and 1 hour's treatment with 28% hydrogen peroxide with supplemental light.[12] A combination technique of in-office bleaching plus home bleaching has been shown to be more effective than in-office bleaching alone.[13] Bernardon and colleagues[14] compared the clinical efficacy of home bleaching, in-office bleaching (with and without light), and a combination technique of in-office bleaching plus home bleaching. The home bleaching was performed with a take-home custom tray using 10% carbamide peroxide worn for 8 hours a day for 2 weeks. The in-office bleaching was performed using 35% hydrogen peroxide for two, 45-minute sessions, whereas the combination technique was performed with one, 45-minute session with supplemental light followed by home bleaching. Color measurements after the first week showed better bleaching results with in-office bleaching with light or the combination technique compared with the at-home bleaching alone. After 2 weeks, there was no significant difference among the 3 techniques. Realistic expectations should also be set about the final whitening effect, and the patient should be informed that the immediate outcome may be lighter at the outset and rebound to some extent within the first week. If the dentist prescribes a combination technique with which the patient begins to supplement the in-office treatment with at-home bleaching, then the patient may not experience the rebound effect. Postoperative instructions may include a recommendation to wait a minimum of 6 hours after in-office bleaching before drinking any chromogenic drinks.[15]

POTENTIAL SOURCES OF VARIABILITY ASSOCIATED WITH BLEACHING LIGHT STUDIES

Whitening with supplemental lighting is a controversial topic in dentistry not limited to safety-related issues in nondental settings but also because of the conflicting reports published in the existing dental literature.[16] Various types of lasers (argon, CO_2, diode, potassium titanyl phosphate) have been investigated in vitro; some[17–20] report improved bleaching results, whereas others[10,21,22] report no significant effect. A common concern with the use of lasers for bleaching is the potential dangers associated with increased pulpal temperature.[23,24]

Table 1 is a representative sample of the clinical research that has been reported in the dental literature and shows the research variability that exists for bleaching studies using adjunct light. As was noted earlier regarding in vitro studies, the table illustrates the same conflicting evidence on the effects of bleaching light with various in vivo studies. Accordingly, studies reported that some lights were not effective[25,26] and some were effective,[27,28] whereas others[6,29–31] reported variable outcomes resulting from different peroxide formulas, light sources, and shade-evaluation and color-monitoring variables.

Variability Associated with Shade-evaluation and Color-measuring Instruments

The reported effects of bleaching lights are dependent on the accuracy and repeatability of the shade-evaluation and color-measuring tools used in a given study. Improvements in color change are typically measured using either visual or instrumental methods, or preferably a combination of the two.

The visual method involves recording baseline tooth shades using dental shade guides compared with after bleaching treatment effects. The most common shade guide used in bleaching studies is the Vitapan Classical Shade Guide (Vita Zahnfabrik, Bad Säckingen, Germany). The shade tabs are arranged from lightest to darkest according to the so-called value-ordered arrangement recommended by the manufacturer. However, the inherent flaws of the Vita Classical Shade Guide in regards to its lack of uniformity, and limited color-space coverage of natural teeth, are well established.[32–35] According to the value-ordered scale, the results of a shade improvement from B3 to D2 are recorded as a change of 7 shade-guide units; however, the shade guide is not specifically designed for evaluating bleaching results and lacks a true value order. Spectrophotometric measurements of the Vita Classical Shade Guide show the nonlinear order of this shade guide, which is frequently used in bleaching studies (**Fig. 4**).[36]

One study compared the effects of a bleaching light using a shade guide designed specifically for monitoring tooth bleaching (Vita Bleachedguide 3D-Master, Vita Zahnfabrik, Bad Säckingen, Germany) and showed a significant effect with a true value-scale shade guide, whereas no difference could be detected using the Vita Classical Shade Guide.[6] Because of the uneven color distribution associated with the Vita Classical Shade Guide, it is possible that real color differences that exist may not be determined using this scale.

Various instrumental methods for measuring color are used in dentistry, such as colorimeters, spectrophotometers, and to a lesser extent imaging systems such as digital cameras.[37] A concern with the use of digital cameras is the calibration for color and the reproducibility among researchers.[38] Colorimeters are considered less reliable and potentially less accurate than spectrophotometers because of aging filters.[39] One critical issue with all these color-measuring instruments is the repeatability of the instrument. Increased variability can be introduced with hand-held intraoral instruments being placed too close to the incisal edge, increasing the transmission of light,[40] or angulations of the instrument, leading to the scattering of light from the face of the aperture (edge loss). To control for deviations in instrument placement, a custom alignment device should be used in research studies to allow for repeatable positioning of the instrument aperture.

Variability Associated with Different Light Sources

Although the popular consumer term for in-office bleaching with light is often referred to as laser bleaching, the more common light source used for bleaching is

Table 1
Variables associated with clinical bleaching light studies

References	Light Efficacious	Timing of Color Comparison	Bleach Concentration Application Time	Light Source — Type	Light Source — Spectrum (nm)	Light Source — Power	Visual Method — Type	Visual Method — Shade Taking Light	Instrumental Method — Consensus	Instrumental Method — Equipment	Instrumental Method — Repeatability	Comments
Papathanasiou et al, 2002[26]	No	24 h	35% HP, 20 min	Halogen curing light	Not reported	Not reported	Vital Classical	Not reported	Yes 3 evaluators	NA	NA	35% of the subjects showed improvement with the light initially
Hein et al, 2003[25]	No	Immediate 1 wk	35% HP, 24 min 38% HP, 60 min 25% HP, 60 min	Xenon-halogen lamp Halogen curing light Metal halide lamp	405–580 440–528 362–587	65 mW/cm 128 mW/cm 72 mW/cm	Vita 3D-Master nonlinear	5500 K Room lights	Not reported 3 evaluators	NA	NA	Unconventional shade-scoring method No significant effect with light was reported for all lights Only 5 patients per group
Tavares et al, 2003[27]	Yes	Immediate 3 mo 6 mo	15% HP, 60 min	Metal halide lamp	400–505	130–160 wW/cm²	Vita Classical	Full-spectrum Operatory light	No	Colorimeter	Custom stent	A significant effect with light was reported with the instrumental method immediately, but no probability value was reported beyond this time or for visual method
Ziemba et al, 2005[28]	Yes	Immediate 1 wk 1 mo	20% HP, 45 min	Metal halide lamp	365–500	Not reported	Vita Classical	5500 K Room lights	No	NA	NA	A significant effect with lights was reported immediately and after 1 week. After 1 month the light group was better but to a significant level

Study				Light source			Shade guide			Instrument		Results
Kugal et al, 2006[31]	Variable	Immediate 2 wk	15% HP, 60 min 38% HP, 60 min	Metal halide lamp	Not reported	Not reported	Vita Classical	5500 K Room lights	Yes 2 evaluators	Digital photography Adobe Photoshop	Not reported	A significant effect with light was reported with the instrumental method, but not after 2 weeks and not with the shade guide
Gurgan et al, 2009[30]	Variable	1 wk	37% HP, 8 min 35% HP, 60 min 38% HP, 30–40 min	Diode laser Light-emitting diode Plasma arc light	815 400–500 400–490	10 W Not reported 2800 mV/cm²	Vita Classical	No	No	Spectrophotometer	Not reported	A significant effect with light was reported with the instrumental method with the diode laser but not with the shade guide
Ontiveros et al, 2009[6]	Variable	1 wk	28% HP, 45 min	Metal halide lamp	350–600	25 W	Vita Classical Vita Bleached	5500 K RiteLite	Yes 3 evaluators	Spectrophotometer	Custom jig	A significant effect with light was reported with the instrumental method and visual method using the bleached guide but not the classical
Calatayud et al, 2010[29]	Variable	Immediate	35% HP, 20 min	Light-emitting diode	380–530	Not reported	Vita Classical	5500 K Demetron shade light	Yes 3 evaluators	NA	NA	A significant effect with light was reported when grouping results for central incisors, laterals, and canines, but not when evaluated separately

Abbreviations: HP, hydrogen peroxide; NA, not available.

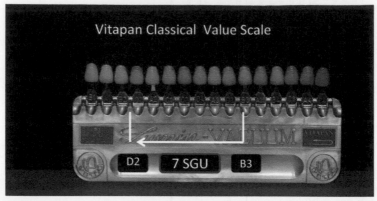

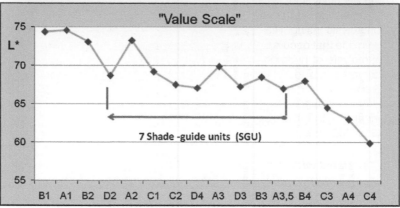

Fig. 4. The Vita Classical Shade Guide arranged by value scale. According to shade tab arrangement, a shade shift from B3 to D2 should be a 7 shade-guide unit change. However, lightness values (L*) from a spectrophotometer show that D2 is darker than B3. (*Data from* Paravina RD, Johnston WM, Powers JM. New shade guide for evaluation of tooth whitening–colorimetric study. J Esthet Restor Dent 2007;19(5):276–83 [discussion: 283].)

high-intensity discharge (HID) lamps (metal halide, xenon arc, plasma arc) or some type of blue light-emitting diode (LED) lamp. An HID lamp is a type of arc lamp that produces light by passing an electric arc through a mixture of gases or metal halides. These lamps are typically wide-spectrum lamps using UV and infrared (IR) filters, narrowing the emission primarily to the violet-blue light spectrum (350–500 nm). The LED lamp is a semiconductor light source capable of producing narrow-spectrum light without the need of filtration.

The use of light as a means of decomposing a chemical compound is known as photolysis. The use of light to assist with the decomposition of hydrogen peroxide was reported in the dental literature as early as 1918.[41] It was commonly accepted that heat was responsible for the dissociation of hydrogen peroxide. Heat was used with some success by heating metal instruments and directly causing an exothermic reaction when applied to the peroxide.[42,43] Direct conductive heat is no longer advocated because of the risk of increasing the pulpal temperature beyond the critical threshold of 5.5°C, which is believed to cause irreversible pulpal damage.[44] It is important that the clinician be familiar with the amount of heat that is generated with the light they choose to use. Caution has been advised regarding increased pulpal temperature, which may increase with some light sources[24] An in vitro bleaching study was conducted in which a xenon arc lamp was compared with a diode laser near IR (960 nm); the study showed that the diode laser produced an unsafe temperature increase up to 12°C beyond the critical threshold. Similar results were reported by Zhang and colleagues[19] with a diode laser near IR (980 nm). Sulieman and colleagues,[45] using a plasma arc lamp, xenon-halogen lamp, halogen lamp, and a diode laser, found the only lamp to produce pulpal temperatures beyond the critical threshold was the diode laser near IR (830 nm). This finding considered, it may not be feasible to rely on photothermal light sources near IR or heat because of the documented risk of increased temperature, which can lead to irreversible pulpitis, and because heat does not seem to be responsible for the dissociation of hydrogen peroxide from certain short-wavelength HID lamps. A photochemical process using short wavelengths may prove to be a preferred approach. Photolysis of hydrogen peroxide can occur by light of wavelengths of 365 nm or less.[46] One study outside dentistry has investigated the effect of various temperatures (15–85°C) on hydrogen peroxide photolysis using HID lamps[47] and concluded that the dissociation of hydrogen peroxide that occurs by lamp irradiation was not dependent on temperature. Although photolysis of hydrogen peroxide was clearly evident, the spectral output lamps were too far into the UV-C range (100–280 nm) to be safe for intraoral use in dentistry. Also, any light with a spectrum in the UV-B range (280–315 nm) is not acceptable for intraoral use. Many of the HID lamps used in dentistry have a spectral emission primarily in the visible spectrum (400–700 nm) and some portions of the UV-A spectrum (315–400 nm).

Variability Associated with Different Lights and Bleaching Formula Interactions

Another variable to consider in light-assisted bleaching is the bleaching formula. A photochemical process can be involved in accelerating the decomposition of peroxide in which light energy with spectral emissions compatible with certain catalytic accelerators/photosensitizes is incorporated into the bleaching formula. Carotenoids, absorbed primarily at wavelengths of 400 to 500 nm, have been used as a bleaching agent activator that also serves as a colorant, giving the otherwise colorless hydrogen peroxide a red-orange color (**Fig. 5**). If the bleaching agent absorbs the light energy of any frequency, it heats and thus decomposes.

Many metals are able to promote oxygen transfer reactions, which enhance the oxidizing power of hydrogen peroxide. These metals include transitional metal

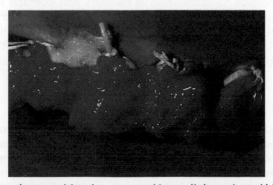

Fig. 5. A red-orange photosensitizer incorporated into a light-activated bleaching to absorb and transfer energy to the peroxide and accelerate decomposition.

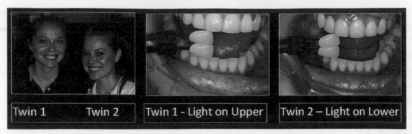

Fig. 6. Identical twins treated with in-office bleaching light. Teeth were treated for 45 minutes using a ferrous activated 38% hydrogen peroxide with and without exposure to an HID lamp. The first twin received light activation on the maxillary teeth and hydrogen peroxide alone on the mandibular teeth 1 week later. The second twin received the opposite treatment: hydrogen peroxide plus light on the mandibular teeth and hydrogen peroxide alone on the maxillary teeth. Slight shade improvements were observed on the teeth activated with the bleaching lamp.

compounds, titanium dioxide, tin oxide, magnesium sulfate, or ferrous compounds. With ferrous compounds, hydrogen peroxide can be combined with iron (II) known as Fenton reagent. Fenton reagents result in disproportion in which the iron is simultaneously reduced and oxidized to form both hydroxyl and peroxide radicals by the same hydrogen peroxide and may occur in the absence or presence of UV light. When Fe^{3+} reacts with UV radiation (photoFenton) the process is renewed and the redox reaction is further fuel:

$$Fe^{2+} + H_2O_2{}^{uv} \rightarrow Fe^{3+} + OH + OH^- \tag{1}$$
$$Fe^{3+} + H_2O_2{}^{uv} \rightarrow Fe^{2+} + OOH\cdot + H^+ \tag{2}$$

Variability Associated with UV Light and Dentinal Absorption

In natural waters, it has been shown that chromophoric dissolved organic matter can undergo photolysis by exposure to UV radiation, leading to the formation of hydrogen peroxide.[48] It has been postulated that UV irradiation of the chromophoric organic matter within the hydrated endogenous dentinal matrix of stained teeth may initiate a similar effect of renewing the hydrogen peroxide during the bleaching process and thus potentiate the bleaching effect.[6] However, further research is required to understand the range of UV light under which the most efficient photolysis occurs with hydrogen peroxide formulas used in dentistry and perhaps within the dental hard tissues themselves. A case of identical twins is presented showing shade improvement on the arch of each twin that was treated with hydrogen peroxide activated with an HID lamp extending in to the UV spectrum. (**Fig. 6**) Although the difference between the light and light arches was not dramatic, it was visually evident to the trained observer.

SUMMARY

Many clinicians use light/indirect radiation to hasten and enhance in-office vital bleaching. What separates the dental professional from the nondental bleach provider is the dental diagnosis and treatment planning required for providing safe and effective treatment. Advantages and disadvantages of different treatment options with realistic expectations for treatment times and outcomes should be a part of the professional consultation.

Clinical studies investigating the use of supplementary light on the effectiveness of vital bleaching have been equivocal. This lack of agreement may result from the variability associated with methods used to measure color, different light sources, and bleaching formula interactions. As new evidence begins to emerge from ongoing research on different bleaching light sources and photochemical interactions of the chromophoric organic matter within natural teeth and catalyzed hydrogen peroxide, we can begin to realize the full benefits of providing safe and effective tooth whitening with adjunct lights.

REFERENCES

1. Wright EP. Bleaching of discolored dentine practically considered. Int Dent J 1890;11(2):70–4.
2. Haywood VB, Heymann HO. Nightguard vital bleaching. Quintessence Int 1989; 20(3):173–6.
3. Hasson H, Ismail AI, Neiva G. Home-based chemically-induced whitening of teeth in adults. Cochrane Database Syst Rev 2006;4:CD006202.
4. Garvin J. Alabama judge rules commercial teeth whitening within dental practice scope. Chicago (IL): American Dental Association, ADA News; 2009.
5. American Dental Association petitions FDA to classify, regulate tooth-whitening products. Chicago (IL): American Dental Association, ADA News; 2009.
6. Ontiveros JC, Paravina RD. Color change of vital teeth exposed to bleaching performed with and without supplementary light. J Dent 2009;37(11):840–7.
7. Haywood VB, Cordero R, Wright K, et al. Brushing with a potassium nitrate dentifrice to reduce bleaching sensitivity. J Clin Dent 2005;16(1):17–22.
8. Haywood VB. Treating sensitivity during tooth whitening. Compend Contin Educ Dent 2005;26(9 Suppl 3):11–20.
9. Charakorn P, Cabanilla LL, Wagner WC, et al. The effect of preoperative ibuprofen on tooth sensitivity caused by in-office bleaching. Oper Dent 2009; 34(2):131–5.
10. Bruzell EM, Johnsen B, Aalerud TN, et al. In vitro efficacy and risk for adverse effects of light-assisted tooth bleaching. Photochem Photobiol Sci 2009;8(3): 377–85.
11. Auschill TM, Hellwig E, Schmidale S, et al. Efficacy, side-effects and patients' acceptance of different bleaching techniques (OTC, in-office, at-home). Oper Dent 2005;30(2):156–63.
12. da Costa JB, McPharlin R, Paravina RD, et al. Comparison of at-home and in-office tooth whitening using a novel shade guide. Oper Dent 2010;35(4):381–8.
13. Matis BA, Cochran MA, Wang G, et al. A clinical evaluation of two in-office bleaching regimens with and without tray bleaching. Oper Dent 2009;34(2):142–9.
14. Bernardon JK, Sartori N, Ballarin A, et al. Clinical performance of vital bleaching techniques. Oper Dent 2010;35(1):3–10.
15. Ontiveros JC, Eldiwany MS, Benson B. Time dependent influence of stain exposure following power bleaching. J Dent Res 2008;87(Spec Iss B):1083.
16. Buchalla W, Attin T. External bleaching therapy with activation by heat, light or laser–a systematic review. Dent Mater 2007;23(5):586–96.
17. Lima DA, Aguiar FH, Liporoni PC, et al. In vitro evaluation of the effectiveness of bleaching agents activated by different light sources. J Prosthodont 2009;18(3): 249–54.
18. Dostalova T, Jelinkova H, Housova D, et al. Diode laser-activated bleaching. Braz Dent J 2004;15(Spec No):SI3–8.

19. Zhang C, Wang X, Kinoshita J, et al. Effects of KTP laser irradiation, diode laser, and LED on tooth bleaching: a comparative study. Photomed Laser Surg 2007; 25(2):91–5.

20. Wetter NU, Barroso MC, Pelino JE. Dental bleaching efficacy with diode laser and LED irradiation: an in vitro study. Lasers Surg Med 2004;35(4):254–8.

21. Gomes MN, Francci C, Medeiros IS, et al. Effect of light irradiation on tooth whitening: enamel microhardness and color change. J Esthet Restor Dent 2009; 21(6):387–94.

22. Wetter NU, Walverde D, Kato IT, et al. Bleaching efficacy of whitening agents activated by xenon lamp and 960-nm diode radiation. Photomed Laser Surg 2004; 22(6):489–93.

23. Luk K, Tam L, Hubert M. Effect of light energy on peroxide tooth bleaching. J Am Dent Assoc 2004;135(2):194–201 [quiz: 228–9].

24. Baik JW, Rueggeberg FA, Liewehr FR. Effect of light-enhanced bleaching on in vitro surface and intrapulpal temperature rise. J Esthet Restor Dent 2001;13(6): 370–8.

25. Hein DK, Ploeger BJ, Hartup JK, et al. In-office vital tooth bleaching–what do lights add? Compend Contin Educ Dent 2003;24(4A):340–52.

26. Papathanasiou A, Kastali S, Perry RD, et al. Clinical evaluation of a 35% hydrogen peroxide in-office whitening system. Compend Contin Educ Dent 2002;23(4): 335–8, 40, 43–4 passim [quiz: 348].

27. Tavares M, Stultz J, Newman M, et al. Light augments tooth whitening with peroxide. J Am Dent Assoc 2003;134(2):167–75.

28. Ziemba SL, Felix H, MacDonald J, et al. Clinical evaluation of a novel dental whitening lamp and light-catalyzed peroxide gel. J Clin Dent 2005;16(4):123–7.

29. Calatayud JO, Calatayud CO, Zaccagnini AO, et al. Clinical efficacy of a bleaching system based on hydrogen peroxide with or without light activation. Eur J Esthet Dent 2010;5(2):216–24.

30. Gurgan S, Cakir FY, Yazici E. Different light-activated in-office bleaching systems: a clinical evaluation. Lasers Med Sci 2009;25(6):817–22.

31. Kugel G, Papathanasiou A, Williams AJ 3rd, et al. Clinical evaluation of chemical and light-activated tooth whitening systems. Compend Contin Educ Dent 2006; 27(1):54–62.

32. Sproull RC. Color matching in dentistry. I. The three-dimensional nature of color. J Prosthet Dent 1973;29(4):416–24.

33. Haywood VB. Color Measurement Symposium 2003. J Esthet Restor Dent 2003; 15(Suppl 1):S3–4.

34. Miller L. Organizing color in dentistry. J Am Dent Assoc 1987;(Spec No):26E–40E.

35. Browning WD. Use of shade guides for color measurement in tooth-bleaching studies. J Esthet Restor Dent 2003;15(Suppl 1):S13–20.

36. Paravina RD, Johnston WM, Powers JM. New shade guide for evaluation of tooth whitening–colorimetric study. J Esthet Restor Dent 2007;19(5):276–83 [discussion: 283].

37. Paravina RD, Powers JM. Esthetic color training in dentistry. 1st edition. St Louis (MO): Elsevier Mosby; 2004.

38. Ishikawa-Nagai S, Terui T, Ishibashi K, et al. Comparison of effectiveness of two 10% carbamide peroxide tooth-bleaching systems using spectrophotometric measurements. J Esthet Restor Dent 2004;16(6):368–75 [discussion: 375–6].

39. Kim-Pusateri S, Brewer JD, Davis EL, et al. Reliability and accuracy of four dental shade-matching devices. J Prosthet Dent 2009;101(3):193–9.

40. Chu SJ, Trushkowsky RD, Paravina RD. Dental color matching instruments and systems. Review of clinical and research aspects. J Dent 2010;38(Suppl 2): e2–16.

41. Abbot CH. Bleaching discolored teeth by means of 30% perhydrol and the electric light rays. J Allied Dent Society 1918;13:259.

42. Hodosh M, Mirman M, Shklar G, et al. A new method of bleaching discolored teeth by the use of a solid state direct heating device. Dent Dig 1970;76(8):344–6.

43. Chandra S, Chawla TN. Clinical evaluation of heat method for bleaching of discoloured mottled teeth. J Indian Dent Assoc 1974;46(8):313–8.

44. Zach L, Cohen G. Pulp response to externally applied heat. Oral Surg Oral Med Oral Pathol 1965;19:515–30.

45. Sulieman M, MacDonald E, Rees JS, et al. Comparison of three in-office bleaching systems based on 35% hydrogen peroxide with different light activators. Am J Dent 2005;18(3):194–7.

46. Baxendale J, Wilson J. The photolysis of hydrogen peroxide at high light intensities. Trans Faraday Soc 1957;52(B):344–56.

47. Garcia Einschlag F, Feliz M, Capparelli A. Effect of temperature on hydrogen peroxide photolysis in aqueous solution. J Photochem Photobiol A Chem 1997; 110:235–42.

48. Del Vecchio R, Blough NV. Photobleaching of chromophoric dissolved organic matter in natural waters: kinetics and modeling. Mar Chem 2002;78:231–53.

Safety Controversies in Tooth Bleaching

Yiming Li, DDS, MSD, PhD[a,b,]*

KEYWORDS

• Peroxide • Safety • Toxicity • Tooth bleaching

In-office tooth bleaching has been a dental procedure for more than a century; however, at-home tooth bleaching was not available until 1989, when it was introduced by Haywood and Heymann.[1,2] With its demonstrated efficacy, lower cost than in-office bleaching, and the convenience of self-application, at-home bleaching quickly gained popularity and has now become an integrated procedure in aesthetic dentistry.[3] Nowadays, in addition to the bleaching products available from dental professionals, over-the-counter (OTC) and infomercial at-home bleaching products are available directly to consumers, and they can be applied with a custom or preformed tray, with a brush, or as a strip. In recent years, tooth bleaching similar to in-office procedures but performed under nondental settings, such as mall kiosks, spas, and cruise ships, has become available.[4]

Current tooth bleaching materials, whether used in office or at home, almost exclusively use peroxide compounds as the active ingredient, with carbamide peroxide and hydrogen peroxide (H_2O_2) being the most common.[2,5] Chemically, carbamide peroxide is composed of approximately 3.5 parts of H_2O_2 and 6.5 parts of urea, so that a bleaching material of 10% carbamide peroxide contains approximately 3.5% H_2O_2. Attempts were made to introduce at-home whiteners that claimed to contain no peroxide; however, such products did not gain acceptance because of the lack of evidence on their efficacy and controversy over their nonperoxide claim.[5] Typically, H_2O_2 concentrations of in-office bleaching products range from 25% to 38%, whereas at-home formulations contain 3.0% to 7.5% H_2O_2. However, in the recent years, there has been a trend of elevating the H_2O_2 concentration in at-home bleaching materials, and products containing up to 15% H_2O_2 have now become available directly to consumers for home use.

The efficacy of peroxide-containing tooth bleaching products has been debated. In general, data accumulated over the last 2 decades also suggest that tooth bleaching is

The author has nothing to disclose.
a Center for Dental Research, Loma Linda University School of Dentistry, 24876 Taylor Street, Loma Linda, CA 92350, USA
b Department of Microbiology and Molecular Genetics, Loma Linda University School of Medicine, Loma Linda, CA, USA
* Center for Dental Research, Loma Linda University School of Dentistry, 24876 Taylor Street, Loma Linda, CA 92350.
E-mail address: yli@llu.edu

Dent Clin N Am 55 (2011) 255–263
doi:10.1016/j.cden.2011.01.003
0011-8532/11/$ – see front matter © 2011 Elsevier Inc. All rights reserved.

a relatively safe procedure. However, controversy concerning its safety has continued since the introduction of the home-use materials, and there have been reports of adverse effects of bleaching on oral tissues and restorative materials.[6–10] This article provides an overview of safety controversies in bleaching in relation to the biologic properties of H_2O_2 and discusses the proper use of bleaching to maximize benefits while minimizing potential risks.

BIOLOGICAL PROPERTIES OF H_2O_2 AND SAFETY CONCERNS WITH BLEACHING

H_2O_2 is a well-investigated chemical. It was discovered in 1818 and detected in human respiration in 1880. The well-known Fenton reaction was proposed in 1894. Peroxidase and catalase, which are 2 important enzymes in H_2O_2 metabolism, were discovered in 1898 and 1901, respectively. Shortly after the discovery of another enzyme, superoxide dismutase (SOD), in 1969, H_2O_2 was recognized as an important byproduct in oxygen metabolism, and the research efforts on the biologic properties of H_2O_2 have been significantly increased since then.[2]

H_2O_2 is a normal intermediate metabolite in the human body, with a daily production of approximately 6.48 g in the liver. One of the key characteristics of H_2O_2 is its capability of producing free radicals, including hydroxyl radicals that have been implicated in various stages of carcinogenesis. Oxidative reactions of free radicals with proteins, lipids, and nucleic acids are thought to be involved in several potential pathologic consequences; the damage by oxidative free radicals may be associated with aging, stroke, and other degenerative diseases.[11,12] To prevent potential damage to cells during oxidative reactions and repair any damage sustained, there are various defensive mechanisms available at cellular and tissue levels. Enzymes such as catalase, SOD, peroxidase, and selenium-dependent glutathione peroxidase, which exist widely in body fluids, tissues, and organs, effectively metabolize H_2O_2.[13] Human saliva also contains these enzymes. In fact, salivary peroxidase has been suggested to be the body's most important and effective defense against the potential adverse effects of H_2O_2.[14] A study on infants, juveniles, adults, and adults with impaired salivary flow found rapid decomposition of H_2O_2 in dentifrices.[15] After brushing for 1 minute with 1 g dentifrice, less than 2% of the prebrushing dose of H_2O_2 (30 mg) was detectable in the oral cavity of the subjects.

Much of the safety concerns with home-use bleaching originate from H_2O_2 used in the materials, especially the known toxicology of free radicals. The oxidative reactions and subsequent damage in cells caused by free radicals are thought to be the major mechanisms responsible for the observed toxicity of H_2O_2. There have been concerns of potential systemic adverse effects if the bleaching material is ingested as well as local adverse effects on enamel, pulp, and gingiva because of the direct contact of the material with the tissues.[2] The safety controversies over peroxide-based tooth bleaching have prompted not only scientific deliberations but also legal challenges to its use in dentistry.[16,17]

CONCERNS WITH SYSTEMIC EFFECTS OF H_2O_2 IN BLEACHING

Considering the dosage and application mode of tooth bleaching, the exposure to the material during the bleaching procedure is inadequate to cause acute systemic toxicity. Although H_2O_2 is found to be mutagenic in the in vitro Ames test without S9 rat liver microsomes, it is not genotoxic in the same test when S9 is incorporated; it is not genotoxic in various animal models either.[2]

With the available data on the toxicity of H_2O_2 as well as the research on bleaching materials and the assessment of their exposure in bleaching, concerns with potential systemic health risks have largely diminished, including the acute, subacute, and chronic toxicities associated with the use of materials containing 10% carbamide peroxide. This reduction is mainly because H_2O_2 exposure from bleaching is limited to the oral cavity and is incapable of reaching a systemic level. The possible exposure dose of H_2O_2 has been estimated at approximately 3.5 mg for a treatment of both arches with a whitener containing 10% carbamide peroxide,[2] whereas the oral cavity is capable of decomposing more than 29 mg H_2O_2 within 1 minute.[15]

CONTROVERSY OVER CARCINOGENICITY OF H_2O_2 IN BLEACHING

The issue of carcinogenicity of H_2O_2 is controversial in the literature, and the published results are contradictory in some studies.[17] Most studies found no evidence of carcinogenicity of H_2O_2; a few showed that H_2O_2 was anticarcinogenic, whereas several reported carcinogenicity or cocarcinogenicity of H_2O_2. The studies that have been cited most frequently as the evidence of carcinogenicity and cocarcinogenicity of H_2O_2 were reported by Ito and colleagues[18–20] and Weitzman and colleagues.[21] However, evaluation of these studies found significant deficiencies in design and conduct of the experiments as well as in the assessment of the results; consequently, the findings of these 4 studies were determined to be inadequate to substantiate their conclusions.[17]

It is obvious that the carcinogenic and cocarcinogenic potential of a tooth bleaching agent constitutes a significant health risk. Because of the potential significance of the study by Weitzman and colleagues,[21] which used local application of H_2O_2 on the oral mucosa of Syrian golden hamsters, the same study was repeated using proper design and methods; the results found no evidence of carcinogenicity or cocarcinogenicity of 3% H_2O_2.[22] Consequently, bleaching using 10% carbamide peroxide is regarded to be of no significant carcinogenic or cocarcinogenic risks. The overall data on bleaching obtained from more than 20 years also seem to support this conclusion. However, because of the significance of the carcinogenicity and relatively limited data available on the topic for bleaching, questions and debates over the carcinogenic risks of bleaching arise periodically. Future research is encouraged to help clarify the controversy and concerns with the topic.

POTENTIAL LOCAL ADVERSE EFFECTS ASSOCIATED WITH BLEACHING

Tooth bleaching requires direct contact of the material with the enamel surface. Although the gingival contact with the bleaching material is not intended, it often occurs when the material is applied at home by consumers. For some at-home systems, such as strips, the gingival contact is inevitable. Some bleaching regimens also involve a continued contact period of up to 7 to 8 hours (overnight). Consequently, possible adverse effects of bleaching on the enamel, pulp, and gingiva have been suggested and investigated.

Potential Adverse Effects on Enamel

The effects of bleaching on enamel were primarily examined in vitro using extracted human or bovine teeth. Bleaching seems to have minimal or no effects on enamel microhardness and mineral content; however, the results on enamel surface change are inconsistent.[23–26] Most scanning electron microscopic studies showed little or no morphologic changes of enamel surfaces associated with bleaching, whereas several studies reported significant alteration of enamel surfaces, including depression, porosity, and erosion, after bleaching. In most cases, however, the observed enamel surface alterations varied with the bleaching products used and seemed to be associated with those patients using acidic prerinse or gels of low pH. The clinical relevancy of the observed changes in the enamel surface morphology has also been questioned. Studies have shown that some soft drinks and fruit juices are capable of causing comparable or greater demineralization and surface alteration of the enamel than those reported for bleaching agents.[26] To date, no clinical evidence of adverse effects of professional at-home bleaching systems on enamel has been reported; however, there have been 2 clinical cases of significant enamel damage associated with the use of OTC bleaching products.[6,7]

Potential Adverse Effects on Gingiva

H_2O_2 at high concentrations is an irritant and also cytotoxic.[2] In cell culture experiments, H_2O_2 is cytotoxic at concentrations ranging from 1.7 to 19.7 µg/mL (0.05–0.58 mmol/L).[27,28] At concentrations of 10% or more, H_2O_2 is potentially corrosive to the mucous membranes or skin, causing a burning sensation and tissue damage.[29] Studies also reported that commercial peroxide-based gels induced cytotoxicity.[29–32]

During the in-office bleaching procedure, which routinely involves the use of H_2O_2 at a concentration of 25% or more, adequate barriers are necessary to protect the gingiva from mucosal damage. If a leakage exists, serious tissue burn can occur. Because of this potential risk, local anesthesia should not be used for in-office bleaching, so that the patient can alert the dentist when the gel seeps through the barriers to cause a burning sensation or pain. However, simply relying on the patient's response is inadequate; clear instructions to the patient to report any discomfort, careful examination of the seal of the barrier after the gel application, and frequent monitoring of the seal throughout the bleaching process are all necessary to minimize the risk of gingival damage and irritation.

Gingival irritation is also common in at-home tooth bleaching. A study[33] found a higher (33.3%) prevalence of gingival irritation in patients using strips of 6.5% H_2O_2 compared with those using at-home tray bleaching with 10% carbamide peroxide (3.5% H_2O_2). A separate study[34] found that 50% of patients using the 6.5% H_2O_2 strips reported gingival irritation, which was about 3 times of those using the 5.3% strips (16.7%). These data indicate that the risk of gingival irritation in at-home bleaching is associated with the H_2O_2 concentration in the bleaching gel, that is, there is a higher prevalence of gingival irritation while using bleaching gels of higher peroxide concentrations. In most cases, the gingival irritation is mild to moderate, tends to be transient, and dissipates when the application discontinues. So far, studies on professional at-home bleaching reported no significant or permanent gingival damage.

Potential Adverse Effects on Pulp and the Risk of Tooth Sensitivity

Recent research, most of which used in vitro models, has shown that H_2O_2 in the bleaching gel applied on the enamel surface is capable of penetrating through the enamel and dentin to reach the pulp chamber.[35–39] An amount of less than 30 µg H_2O_2 may reach the pulp after the application of gels containing up to 12% H_2O_2 on the enamel surface for up to 7 hours. Although the amount of H_2O_2 detected in the pulp chamber tends to increase with the time and H_2O_2 concentration in the gel, such a relationship is not proportional. It was suggested that an amount of 50,000 µg H_2O_2 would be needed to inhibit pulpal enzymes,[40] so the detected amount of H_2O_2 that penetrated into the pulp chamber seems unlikely to cause significant damage to pulp tissues. However, there is a lack of in vivo studies on this topic, and long-term effects of such H_2O_2 exposure on pulp are yet to be determined.

Tooth sensitivity to temperature changes is a commonly observed clinical side effect in bleaching, and it has been suggested as an indication of possible pulp response to H_2O_2 that penetrates through the tooth hard tissue and reaches the pulp, although its mechanisms are not fully understood. Tooth sensitivity may or may not occur with gingival irritation.[41] In some cases, the patient may mistake gingival irritation for tooth sensitivity, or vice versa; therefore, careful examination and differential diagnosis are necessary for appropriate treatment regimens.

In general, up to 1 in 2 people may experience temporary tooth sensitivity as a result of tooth bleaching.[41–44] The development of tooth sensitivity does not seem to be related to the patient's age or sex, defective restorations, enamel-cementum abrasion, or the dental arch treated; however, the risk increases in patients with the frequency of daily application. The incidence and severity of the sensitivity may also depend on the quality of the bleaching material, the techniques used, and an individual's response to the bleaching treatment methods.[4] The sensitivity, usually mild and transient, often occurs during the early stages of tooth whitening, and for most patients it is tolerable to complete the treatment. So far, there are no reported cases of pulp necrosis caused by tooth bleaching; however, teeth with caries, with exposed dentin, in close proximity to pulp horns, or suspected to have cracks are potentially at risk for developing severe sensitivity and thus are not advisable for bleaching. In addition, defective restorations should be replaced before bleaching, and extra caution should be applied to children and adolescents because of their relatively larger pulp chamber.[45]

Potential Adverse Effects on Restorative Materials

Numerous studies have reported that tooth bleaching may adversely affect physical and/or chemical properties of restorative materials, including increased surface roughness, crack development, marginal breakdown, release of metallic ions, and decreased tooth-to-restoration bond strength. Potential adverse effects of bleaching on bonding strength have been well recognized.[9,46,47] A plausible mechanism is the inhibition of adequate polymerization of the bonding agent by the residual oxygen formed during bleaching. Similar effects are also applicable to other resin-based restorative materials that require in situ polymerization. The post-bleaching inhibitory effects on polymerization dissipate with time, and an interval of 2 weeks is found to be adequate to avoid such adverse effects.

A relevant safety concern is the mercury release from amalgam restorations during and after bleaching.[48–50] Although not much debate exists regarding whether bleaching causes mercury release, the reported amount of mercury release associated with bleaching varies greatly. The issue on potential health implications of the mercury released remains controversial and yet to be determined. Because of the known toxicity of mercury, as a general rule, it is not advisable to perform bleaching for those whose teeth are restored extensively with amalgam.

SAFETY CONCERNS WITH BLEACHING WITH NO INVOLVEMENT OF DENTAL PROFESSIONALS

Largely because of the clinically visible efficacy of at-home bleaching, an ever increasing number of OTC home bleaching products have become available directly to consumers shortly after the introduction of the night guard tray bleaching that was originally performed by dental professionals. There are various forms of these OTC bleaching products, including gels applied using a tray or paint-on brush, mouth rinses, chewing gums, toothpastes, and strips. Similar products are also available through infomercials and the internet. More recently, tooth bleaching has become available in mall kiosks, salons, spas, and even cruise ships, which usually simulate the in-office bleaching settings, often involving the use of light but being performed by individuals with no formal dental training and not licensed to practice dentistry. This practice has come under scrutiny in several states and jurisdictions, resulting in actions to reserve the delivery of this service to dentists or appropriately supervised allied dental personnel.[4]

Basically, no scientific research is available on bleaching performed at mall kiosks, salons, spas, and cruise ships, whereas a significant amount of clinical data on the OTC bleaching products are available in the literature.[5,33,34,43] Overall, data indicate that adverse effects associated with the use of OTC bleaching products seem to be rare. There have been only 2 reports on irreversible enamel damage caused by OTC bleaching products.[6,7] However, it is unclear whether the low incidence of adverse effects associated with the use of the OTC bleaching products is the result of their low risk or the lack of means to detect and report adverse effects. The data available in the literature were collected from studies conducted by dental professionals, which were not intended for these OTC products. In addition, consumers are not generally aware of how to report adverse events through the US Food and Drug Administration's MedWatch system.[4] It is a reasonable assumption that when an individual purchases and uses an OTC bleaching product, some adverse effects, such as enamel surface changes, may go unnoticed; even those effects felt or detected by the user remain most likely unreported. More of a concern is the tendency of overusing or abusing an OTC bleaching product. Research efforts are encouraged to define the risks of OTC bleaching products, if any, under relevant scenarios intended for these products.

ROLES OF DENTAL PROFESSIONALS IN TOOTH BLEACHING

It is highly recommended that tooth bleaching involves dental professionals. Initial evaluation and examination of tooth discoloration are necessary for proper diagnosis and treatment; bleaching materials can affect restorative materials and may also result in color mismatch of teeth with existing restorations or crowns. Such evaluations cannot be performed or determined by consumers themselves or nondental individuals. Discoloration, particularly intrinsic stains, may not simply be an aesthetic problem,[5,51] and bleaching may not be the appropriate or the best choice for treatment. For at-home bleaching using trays, professionally fabricated, custom-fit trays reduce the amount of gel needed for maximal efficacy while minimizing the gel contact with gingiva. In addition, periodic evaluation of bleaching progress by dentists allows early detection of any possible side effects and reduces the risk of using poor-quality bleaching materials, inappropriate application procedures, and any temptation to overuse or abuse the product. The American Dental Association encourages all patients interested in tooth bleaching to seek advice from a dental professional.[4,52]

SUMMARY

Tooth bleaching is intended for improving tooth color and has become an accepted and popular dental procedure in aesthetic dentistry. Data accumulated over the last 20 years also indicate no significant, long-term oral or systemic health risks associated with professional at-home tooth bleaching using materials containing 10% carbamide peroxide, which is equivalent to 3.5% H_2O_2.

However, as with any dental procedure, bleaching involves risks. Tooth sensitivity and gingival irritation can occur in a significant portion of the patients, although in most cases they are mild to moderate and transient. When gels of high H_2O_2 concentrations, such as those for in-office bleaching, are used without adequate gingival protection, severe mucosal damage can occur. Although rare, potential adverse effects are possible with inappropriate application, abuse, or the use of inappropriate at-home bleaching products. H_2O_2 is capable of producing various toxic effects, so that potential risks exist and need to be recognized. So far, little data are available on the safety of OTC at-home bleaching that simulates the intended application mode of these products, and the safety of bleaching performed at mall kiosks, salons, spas, and cruise ships is of particular concern because the procedure is similar to that of in-office bleaching but performed by nondental individuals.

Effective and safe tooth bleaching requires correct diagnosis of the problems associated with tooth discoloration or stains. Furthermore, tooth sensitivity and gingival irritation may occur during the course of bleaching treatment. To minimize risks and maximize benefits, the involvement of dental professionals in bleaching treatment is necessary.

REFERENCES

1. Haywood VB, Heymann HO. Nightguard vital bleaching. Quintessence Int 1989; 20:173–6.
2. Li Y. Biological properties of peroxide-containing tooth whiteners. Food Chem Toxicol 1996;34:887–904.
3. Kihn PW. Vital tooth whitening. Dent Clin North Am 2007;51:319–31.
4. American Dental Association (ADA). Tooth whitening/bleaching: treatment considerations for dentists and their patients. Chicago: ADA Council on Scientific Affairs; 2009.
5. Li Y. The safety of peroxide-containing at-home tooth whiteners. Compendium 2003;24:384–9.
6. Cubbon T, Ore D. Hard tissue and home tooth whiteners. CDS Rev 1991;84:32–5.
7. Hammel S. Do-it-yourself tooth whitening is risky. US News and World Report. April 2, 1998;66.
8. Dahl JE, Pallesen U. Tooth bleaching—a critical review of the biological aspects. Crit Rev Oral Biol Med 2003;14:292–304.
9. Attin T, Hannig C, Wiegand A, et al. Effect of bleaching on restorative materials and restorations—a systematic review. Dent Mater 2004;20:852–61.
10. Goldberg M, Grootveld M, Lynch E. Undesirable and adverse effects of tooth-whitening products: a review. Clin Oral Investig 2010;14:1–10.
11. Harman D. The aging process. Proc Natl Acad Sci U S A 1981;78:7124–32.
12. Lutz WK. Endogenous genotoxic agents and processes as a basis of spontaneous carcinogenesis. Mutat Res 1990;238:287–95.
13. Floyd RA. Role of oxygen free radicals in carcinogenesis and brain ischemia. FASEB J 1990;4:2587–97.
14. Carlsson J. Salivary peroxidase: an important part of our defense against oxygen toxicity. J Oral Pathol 1987;16:412–6.
15. Marshall MV, Gragg PP, Packman EW, et al. Hydrogen peroxide decomposition in the oral cavity. Am J Dent 2001;14:39–45.
16. Weiner ML, Freeman C, Trochimowicz H, et al. 13-week drinking water toxicity study of hydrogen peroxide with 6-week recovery period in catalase-deficient mice. Food Chem Toxicol 2000;38:607–15.
17. Li Y. Peroxide-containing tooth whiteners: an update on safety. Compend Contin Educ Dent 2000;21(Suppl 28):S4–9.

18. Ito A, Watanaee H, Naito M, et al. Induction of duodenal tumors in mice by oral administration of hydrogen peroxide. Gann 1981;72:174–5.

19. Ito A, Naito M, Naito Y, et al. Induction and characterization of gastro-duodenal lesions in mice given continuous oral administration of hydrogen peroxide. Gann 1982;73:315–22.

20. Ito A, Watanaee H, Naito M, et al. Correlation between induction of duodenal tumor by hydrogen peroxide and catalase activity in mice. Gann 1984;75:17–21.

21. Weitzman SA, Weitberg AB, Stossel TP, et al. Effects of hydrogen peroxide on oral carcinogenesis in hamsters. J Periodontol 1986;57:685–8.

22. Marshall MV, Kuhn JO, Torrey CF, et al. Hamster cheek pouch bioassay of dentifrices containing hydrogen peroxide and baking soda. J Am Coll Toxicol 1996;15: 45–61.

23. Rotstein I, Li Y. Tooth discoloration and bleaching. In: Ingle JI, Bakland LK, Baumgartner JC, editors. Ingle's endodontics. 6th edition. Hamilton (Canada): BC Decker Inc; 2008. p. 1383–99.

24. Potocnik I, Kosec L, Gaspersic D. Effect of 10% carbamide peroxide bleaching gel on enamel microhardness, microstructure, and mineral content. J Endod 2000;26:203–6.

25. White DJ, Kozak KM, Zoladz JR, et al. Peroxide interactions with hard tissues: effects on surface hardness and surface/subsurface ultrastructural properties. Compend Contin Educ Dent 2002;23:42–8.

26. Ren YF, Amin A, Malmstrom H. Effects of tooth whitening and orange juice on surface properties of dental enamel. J Dent 2009;37:424–31.

27. Grando LJ, Tames DR, Cardoso AC, et al. In vitro study of enamel erosion caused by soft drinks and lemon juice in deciduous teeth analyzed by stereomicroscopy and scanning electron microscopy. Caries Res 1996;30:373–8.

28. Ramp WK, Arnold RR, Russell JE, et al. Hydrogen peroxide inhibits glucose metabolism and collagen synthesis in bone. J Periodontol 1987;58:340–4.

29. Scientific Committee on Consumer Products (European Commission). Opinion on hydrogen peroxide in tooth whitening products. SCCP/0844/04. March 15, 2005.

30. Hanks CT, Fat JC, Wataha JC, et al. Cytotoxicity and dentin permeability of carbamide peroxide and hydrogen peroxide vital bleaching materials, in vitro. J Dent Res 1993;72:931–8.

31. Tse CS, Lynch E, Blake DR, et al. Is home tooth bleaching gel cytotoxic? J Esthet Dent 1991;3:162–8.

32. Woolverton CJ, Haywood VB, Heymann HO. Toxicity of two carbamide peroxide products used in nightguard vital bleaching. Am J Dent 1993;6:310–4.

33. Kugel G, Aboushala A, Zhou X, et al. Daily use of whitening strips on tetracycline-stained teeth: comparative results after 2 months. Compend Contin Educ Dent 2002;23:29–34.

34. Gerlach RW, Zhou X. Comparative clinical efficacy of two professional bleaching systems. Compend Contin Educ Dent 2002;23:35–41.

35. Thitinanthapan W, Satamanont P, Vongsavan N. In vitro penetration of the pulp chamber by three brands of carbamide peroxide. J Esthet Dent 1999;11:259–64.

36. Slezak B, Santarpia P, Xu T, et al. Safety profile of a new liquid whitening gel. Compend Contin Educ Dent 2002;23(Suppl 1):4–11.

37. Benetti AR, Valera MC, Mancini MN, et al. In vitro penetration of bleaching agents into the pulp chamber. Int Endod J 2004;37:120–4.

38. Pugh G, Zaidel L, Lin N, et al. High levels of hydrogen peroxide in overnight tooth-whitening formulas: effects on enamel and pulp. J Esthet Restor Dent 2005;17: 40–5.

39. Camargo SE, Cardoso PE, Valera MC, et al. Penetration of 35% hydrogen peroxide into the pulp chamber in bovine teeth after LED or Nd:YAG laser activation. Eur J Esthet Dent 2009;4:82–8.

40. Bowles WH, Ugwuneri Z. Pulp chamber penetration of hydrogen peroxide following vital bleaching procedures. J Endod 1987;8:875–7.

41. Leonard RH. Efficacy, longevity, side effects, and patient perceptions of night-guard vital bleaching. Compend Contin Educ Dent 1998;19:766–81.

42. Jorgensen MG, Carroll WB. Incidence of tooth sensitivity after home whitening treatment. J Am Dent Assoc 2002;133:1076–82.

43. Hasson H, Ismail AI, Neiva G. Home-based chemically-induced whitening of teeth in adults. Cochrane Database Syst Rev 2006;4:CD006202.

44. Burrows S. A review of the safety of tooth bleaching. Dent Update 2009;36:604–6, 608–10, 612–4.

45. Lee SS, Zhang W, Lee DH, et al. Tooth whitening in children and adolescents: a literature review. Pediatr Dent 2005;27:362–8.

46. Breschi L, Cadenaro M, Antoniolli F, et al. Extent of polymerization of dental bonding systems on bleached enamel. Am J Dent 2007;20:275–80.

47. Lima AF, Fonseca FM, Cavalcanti AN, et al. Effect of the diffusion of bleaching agents through enamel on dentin bonding at different depths. Am J Dent 2010; 23:113–5.

48. Rotstein I, Dogan H, Avron Y, et al. Mercury release from dental amalgam following treatment with 10% carbamide peroxide in vitro. Oral Surg Oral Med Oral Pathol Oral Radiol Endod 2000;89:216–9.

49. Rotstein I, Avron Y, Shemesh H, et al. Factors affecting mercury release from dental amalgam exposed to carbamide peroxide bleaching agent. Am J Dent 2004;17:347–50.

50. Al-Salehi SK. Effects of bleaching on mercury ion release from dental amalgam. J Dent Res 2009;88:239–43.

51. Shafer WG, Hine MG, Levy BM. Textbook of oral pathology. 4th edition. Philadelphia: WB Saunders; 1983. p. 766–8.

52. American Dental Association (ADA). For the dental patient: tooth whitening – what you should know. J Am Dent Assoc 2009;40:384.

Diastema: Correction of Excessive Spaces in the Esthetic Zone

Anabella Oquendo, DDS*, Luis Brea, DDS, Steven David, DMD

KEYWORDS

• Diastema • Excessive space • Dentoalveolar discrepancies
• Closure

The presence of a space, or diastema, between anterior teeth is a common feature of adult dentitions. The spaces usually distort a pleasing smile by concentrating the observer's attention not on the overall dental composition, but on the diastema.[1] However, not every diastema should be viewed by the practitioner as needing correction. The patient's needs, demands, and expectations must be considered in the process of treatment planning to ensure satisfaction with the treatment outcomes.[2]

Many forms of therapy can be used for diastema closure. A carefully developed diagnosis, which includes a determination of the causal elements, and advanced treatment planning, allows the most appropriate treatment to be selected for each case. Explaining the various treatment options to the patient, and documenting their understanding of the options, is critical in gaining the patient's consent and cooperation in achieving a result that will be judged successful.

Orthodontic correction often results in a sensible esthetic improvement and is well accepted by patients. However, orthodontics alone often may not be able to correct the problems associated with excessive space. In many cases, postorthodontic restorative and periodontal procedures are also necessary.[2]

In the past decade, there has been a remarkable upswing in interdisciplinary collaboration between restorative dentists, orthodontists, and periodontists in smile enhancement. As the interactions within the pseudospecialty that has become known as cosmetic dentistry have increased, dentists have become more sensitive to the standards that should guide them in striving to create a more pleasing smile for their patients.[3]

The specific goals of treating diastemata are: creating a tooth form in harmony with adjacent teeth, arch, and facial form; maintaining an environment for excellent gingival health; and attainment of a stable and functional occlusion. The final result should be

Department of Cariology and Comprehensive Care, International Program in Advanced Aesthetic Dentistry, New York University College of Dentistry, 45 East 24 Street, 7W, New York, NY 10010, USA
* Corresponding author.
E-mail address: anabellaop@gmail.com

Dent Clin N Am 55 (2011) 265–281
doi:10.1016/j.cden.2011.02.002
0011-8532/11/$ – see front matter © 2011 Elsevier Inc. All rights reserved.

dental.theclinics.com

one that is harmonious and pleasing to the patient. These goals can be met and clinical success achieved by applying contemporary principles of smile design and following an appropriate sequence of treatment.

CAUSE

Numerous factors contribute to proper tooth and arch interrelationships. These may include the relative height, width, orientation, and the number of teeth as well as the size and shape of the dental arches. An imbalance in size and shape of the teeth and dental arches may limit the ability of the teeth to fit together properly. This may result in the formation of a single or multiple diastemata. It is important to understand the origins of the problem. The significance of any single factor may vary among patients, thus each patient must be evaluated thoroughly before the initiation of any treatment. The causes must always be considered, as they lead to more individualized and effective therapies.[2]

Factors that may be involved in the cause of congenital or acquired diastemata include the following:

- Transition between deciduous and permanent dentition in the normal development of the dentition
- Hereditary or ethnic features
- Enlarged labial frenae
- Regular deleterious behavior (parafunction)
- Unbalanced muscular function
- Physical obstacles
- Defects in the intermaxillary suture
- Accentuated overbite
- Dentoalveolar discrepancies
- Pathologies (eg, partial agenesis, supernumerary teeth, cysts in the anterior region, impeded eruption, palatal cleft)
- Iatrogenic
- Orthodontic mechanics (eg, rapid maxillary expansion, distal movements)
- Anomalies in the shape, size, and number of teeth
- Physiologic or pathologic dental migration
- Tongue and lip habits
- Tooth loss.

Dentoalveolar discrepancies may be listed among the most common causes of anterior diastemata in adults. Dentoalveolar discrepancies usually result from disharmonies between the size of the dental arch and the width of the teeth or from the presence of bone defects that cause diastemata.[2]

CLINICAL CONSIDERATIONS
Esthetic Parameters

A thorough understanding of esthetic principles is also essential in dealing with patients' concerns and demands. Esthetic dentistry is a combination of measurable dimensions and artistic sensitivity.[4] Esthetically the teeth are aligned and related to each other, the surrounding soft tissues, and the patient's facial characteristics. A dynamic, three dimensional blueprint is created that draws attention to the teeth.[5] A systematic esthetic analysis that progresses from facial, dentofacial, dentogingival to dental analysis is mandatory for a successful esthetic outcome of the case.

Tooth Proportion

Achieving ideal tooth shape and proportion is an important goal in diastema correction.[6] An imbalance in the proportion of the anterior teeth is frequently observed after the closure of diastemata. A pleasing width to length tooth proportion is an essential requirement for a favorable esthetic outcome.[7]

Tooth proportion is the relationship between measurements derived from dividing the width of the tooth by its length. A pleasant dental proportion for a maxillary central incisor falls within the range of 75% to 85% (**Fig. 1**). The closer the proportion is to 100% the more square the tooth will appear. As the ratio approaches or is less than 75%, the more rectangular and slender the tooth will appear.

Because the proportion depends on 2 variables, height and width, increasing or decreasing one of the variables produces a desirable or undesirable proportion. Precise measurement during the diastema closure is imperative. Proposed changes in any of the dimensions should be quantified and noted, as the size of the required changes often determines the nature of the treatment to be rendered. Changes in the width of a tooth during diastema closure could affect either the individual tooth proportion, the size and shape of interproximal (embrasure) space, the proportion to the adjacent teeth, or the three-dimensional location of a tooth within the arch.[8]

Tooth to tooth proportion

Tooth to tooth proportion represents another cornerstone of esthetic design when closing diastemata. Several investigators have stressed the importance of order in the composition, applying the same recurring ratio from the central incisor to the first premolar.[9] Some believe that the most harmonious recurrent tooth to tooth ratio is found in the golden proportion. The golden proportion implies that the maxillary central incisor should be approximately 62% wider than the lateral incisor and the lateral incisor should be approximately 62% wider than the mesial aspect of the canine. The first premolar would be 62% of the width value of the canine from the frontal view.

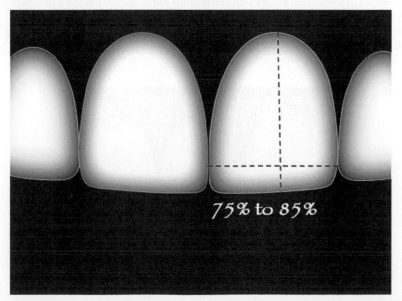

75% to 85%

Fig. 1. A pleasant dental proportion for a maxillary central incisor has a range of 75% to 85%.

However, Chu[10] identified that only 17% of patients fit within these dental ideals and strict adherence to this rule would result in an excessively narrow maxillary arch and compression of the lateral segments.

Ward[9] has described the recurring esthetic dental (RED) proportion stating that the proportion of the successive width of the teeth as viewed from the front should remain constant as one moves distally. Rather than being locked into using the 62% proportion of the golden proportion, the dentist can use a proportion of their own choosing. The RED proportion has been found to be pleasing to patients as well as clinicians, and can be used to arrange the teeth for a pleasing smile.[11] The use of the RED proportion gives more flexibility because it gives the clinician the ability to change the proportions of the teeth to suit the individual patient's face, bone structure, and general physical type.

Chu[10] describes yet another way to relate the width of teeth within the esthetic zone. Chu proposes that the width of the maxillary lateral incisor should be approximately 2 mm less than the central incisor and the width of the canine should be 1 mm less than the central incisor (**Fig. 2**).[12]

Incisal edge position

In addition to addressing space management in the horizontal dimension, vertical tooth position and vertical gingival margin control are important to achieve an ideal restorative result.[6] Evaluating the vertical position of the teeth helps to establish the proper width/length ratio of the clinical crown, and enables the dentist to provide an esthetically pleasing final result.[6]

Optimization of the esthetic outcome of any anterior restoration is primarily determined by the appropriateness of the incisal edge position of the maxillary incisors. This position can be evaluated according to the following parameters.[10]

1. The relationship of the incisal edges with the upper border of the lower lip both at rest and dynamically
2. The length of the incisal edges compared with the length of the buccal cusps of the maxillary posterior teeth
3. The distance between the upper and lower lip
4. The ratio between width and height of the teeth
5. Phonetics.

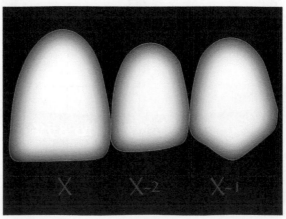

Fig. 2. The width of the maxillary lateral incisor is approximately 2 mm less than the central and the width of the canine is 1 mm less than the central incisor.

Occlusion

Measurement of the horizontal overlap, or overjet, and the vertical overlap, or overbite, convey the horizontal and vertical distances between the upper and lower incisal tables. This relationship influences the esthetic outcome and defines the angle and the anterior component of the envelope of function. All restorations fabricated during treatment must be constructed in harmony with the patient's envelope of function.[12] When considering the correction of an anterior diastema, it is imperative to analyze the affect of the space closure on the function of the stomatognathic system.[5]

Gracis and Chu[11] have suggested a three-step sequence for developing anterior guidance when closing diastemata in the esthetic zone:

1. Determine the incisal edge position (terminal point) through a dentofacial (esthetic) analysis of the patient.
2. Determine the position at which occlusal contact should occur (starting point) at the vertical dimension of occlusion.
3. Develop the intermediate pathway.[10]

Gingival esthetics

The appearance of the teeth and gums must act in concert to provide a balanced and harmonious smile. A defect in the surrounding pink tissues cannot be compensated by the quality of the dental restorations and vice versa.[8]

Gingival Architecture

The gingival outline in the anterior sextant should be symmetric and should vertically align the gingival margin heights of the canines and central incisors. The gingival margin zenith of the lateral incisors should be located approximately 1 mm coronal to the central incisors (**Fig. 3**).[8] The importance of providing gingival symmetry when closing diastemata cannot be overemphasized. The gingival tissues can be altered via periodontal surgery to accomplish an ideal architecture. Resective (ie, gingivectomy, osseous crown lengthening) or additive (ie, gingival grafting, coronal soft tissue reposition) surgeries are recommended when discrepancies in the soft tissue interfere with the proposed tooth proportion or esthetic corrections are necessary.

Altering soft tissue levels can also be accomplished successfully through orthodontic intrusion or extrusion. Among the benefits of the nonsurgical orthodontic approach are preservation of supporting tissues and maintenance of the crown/root ratio. Esthetically, a major advantage is the ability to restore ideal cervical gingival morphology and emergence profile. In addition, the possibility of surgically exposing the root portion of the tooth, with its negative consequences, is eliminated (**Fig. 4**).

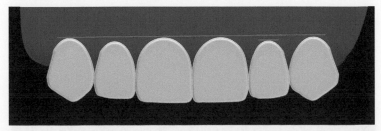

Fig. 3. The progression of the gingival margins (gm) is considered normal when the gm of the lateral incisors is 1 mm coronal to the tangent drawn between the gm of the central incisors and canine.

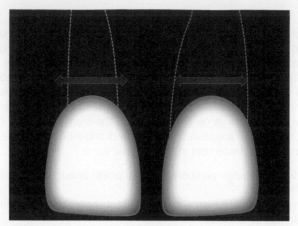

Fig. 4. Altering of the soft tissue levels via surgical procedures is limited by the need to avoid the need for over-contouring the restoration and compromise of cervical gingival morphology and emergence profile.

Location of zenith points is another important consideration in diastema correction. The gingival zenith is defined as the most apical point of the marginal gingiva. Its shape and location is determined by the anatomy and contours of the tooth, the position of the tooth within the arch, enamel extensions, and the health of the soft tissue attachment. Under normal anatomic conditions the location of the zenith point on the central is 1 mm distal to the midline of the tooth and at the midline for the lateral incisor and canine (**Fig. 5**).[13]

Papilla formation

The presence of a diastema is one of the causes of the absence of an interdental papilla. Part of the success of the treatment of a diastema depends on the esthetic integration of soft and hard tissue.[7] The balance between white architecture (teeth) and pink architecture (gums) should be esthetically pleasing and natural. In that context, one of the difficulties encountered in closing a diastema is not leaving an excessively wide gingival embrasure, often referred to as a black triangle.[7] Proper design and location of the contact point is the key requirement in avoiding black triangles. To determine the approximate location of the contact point, measurement of the distance between the crestal bone and the gingival margin has to be accomplished.[7]

Measurements[14] have shown that if the distance from the base of the contact point to the crest of the bone is 5 mm or less, the papilla will fill the embrasure almost 100%

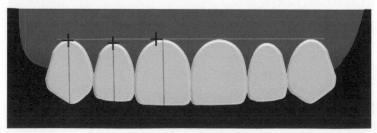

Fig. 5. The location of the zenith point on the central is 1 mm distal to the midline of the tooth and at the midline for the lateral incisor and canine.

of the time. If the distance is 6 mm the papilla will be present only 55% of the time.[15] The importance of these numbers and their usefulness in restoration design cannot be overemphasized. In addition, studies have shown that the papilla proportion for maxillary anterior teeth, as measured from the gingival zenith to the papilla crest, is approximately 40% of the total length of the clinical crown (**Fig. 6**).[16]

TREATMENT OPTIONS

Excessive interproximal space presents a dynamic challenge. Arch circumference or length must be decreased or tooth structure added. Closing spaces exclusively by orthodontics requires that arch length be decreased either by retraction of anterior teeth, protraction of posterior teeth, or a combination of both. Envisioning the end result before adjunctive orthodontics will define the treatment plan.[17] However, treatment plans should not be selected empirically; they should be based on thorough documentation. Measurements, models, and photographs are all parts of adequate treatment planning.

Diastema closure must establish proper tooth proportions that are as close to ideal as possible.[1] Orthodontic intervention alone is not adequate to resolve every problem. When dentoalveolar and Bolton[a] discrepancies are detected, orthodontic intervention is not sufficient to establish the proximal contacts with satisfactory vertical and horizontal overlaps. Restorative intervention is required to optimize results. Orthodontic treatment can be used, however, to redistribute the spaces between the maxillary anterior teeth before the restorative procedures.[18]

The literature documents many methods for treating anterior diastemata: porcelain laminate veneers, direct bonding, and crowns, both with and without orthodontics.[19] Regardless of the treatment chosen, the patient should be aware that along with esthetic improvement there is a concurrent change in speech.[2] The passage of air through the oral cavity during speech will be modified when the diastema is closed. The patient should be advised before initiating treatment that a change in speech may occur. Phonetic evaluation (enunciation of F, S and V sounds) is advised. If there is a change in speech that is noticeable and troublesome, the patient should be advised that adaptation to this new speech pattern usually occurs within a few days.[2] Reading aloud is a useful exercise to help the patient return to previous speech patterns.

ORTHODONTIC APPROACH

A shift from traditional orthodontic treatment goals, such as ideal occlusion and cephalometric standards, to include goals embodying principles of microesthetics and soft tissue harmony has occurred. Orthodontists now place a greater emphasis on gingival esthetics, tooth form, and increasingly rely on interdisciplinary care.[6]

The use of orthodontic treatment alone to close a diastema is most appropriate in those cases in which proximal contacts can be obtained without the use of addition restorations.[2] This is possible when acceptable tooth proportion and tooth size exist.[6] Patients with significant overjet can often be treated with orthodontics alone as closing of the maxillary spaces will reduce the overjet. If, however, a patient does not exhibit excess overjet, closing the space orthodontically, without restorative dentistry, may be detrimental for the functional occlusion because of the possible over-retraction of the incisors.[6] This, almost certainly, will cause multiple long-term problems such as increased occlusal wear on the anterior teeth, crowding of the lower incisors, or

---

[a] A Bolton analysis is a calculation developed by Wayne Bolton for the evaluation of discrepancies in the sum of tooth widths between upper and lower aches.

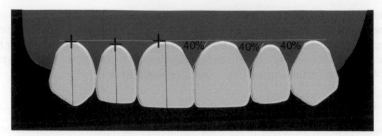

Fig. 6. The papilla to crown length proportion for the maxillary anterior teeth is approximately 40%.

relapse of the spacing. Orthodontic space closure may also lead to a constriction of the anterior arch width and adversely affect smile esthetics.[6]

Although orthodontics is capable of providing a pleasing esthetic result, its major disadvantage is the amount of time and the number of appointments required to obtain the desired esthetic result. In addition, orthodontic relapse may occur without proper retention and stabilization. Fixed orthodontic appliances may result in an increased accumulation of plaque, increasing caries, and periodontal susceptibility. On the other hand, removable orthodontic appliances are effective only if patients comply with instructions. Failing to wear the removable appliance as directed will produce poor results or increase the amount of time needed to obtain the desired results.[19]

When maxillary anterior teeth are not proportional to both mandibular anterior teeth and within the arch, and spaces exist, it is not possible to obtain proximal contacts with orthodontic intervention alone. A restorative approach is required to close the diastema.[2]

Restorative Approach

Direct bonding, laminate veneers, and crowns are used to correct diastemata. These modalities control both tooth size and shape.

Direct

Direct composite resin restorations and direct composite veneers are a conservative therapy that can provide a good treatment outcome in diastema closure. Both esthetics and function are enhanced and, in most cases, little or no preparation of the tooth is required. Contemporary composite materials are esthetic, durable, and affordable, and with longevity of adhesion to enamel that is well documented. Physical and chemical improvements over the years have optimized color stability and improved wear resistance.[2]

Additional benefits of direct bonding include ease of intraoral repair, the ability to sculpt the restoration, lower costs, and completion in a single visit without the need to incur laboratory fees.[19] Another advantage of direct bonding is the ability to modify while the patient is still undergoing orthodontic treatment.

The use of direct composite for diastema closure should be limited to patients with excellent oral hygiene. To discourage plaque retention, and its associated loss of gingival health, it is essential to polish the direct composite restoration to a high gloss. Meticulous oral hygiene of well-polished restorations can prevent adverse periodontal affects of even overcountoured and intrasulcular direct composite restorations.[7]

The main disadvantage of composite resin is the possible need for multiple replacements during the lifetime of the patient. The passage of time is not as kind to composite as it is to porcelain and discoloration or degradation usually develops.[6] Therefore patients should be made aware that the shade and texture of the composite material will probably change with time, and that it may require periodic replacement.[18] Arguably, the surface texture of composite veneers is not as natural in appearance as porcelain. In addition, most practitioners find it harder to create teeth directly in the mouth compared with a technician working at a laboratory bench. If anatomic nuances are not followed, an unesthetic V-shaped diastema closure may result.[19]

Indirect

Diastema closure is one of the most common indications for porcelain laminates veneers.[1] For most patients, veneers allow for the conservation of tooth structure, yet offer optimal esthetics. They afford maximum control in establishing shade, contour, and proportion, and maintain their texture and contour indefinitely. Their glazed surface promotes periodontal health through resistance to plaque adherence. However, their cost may be a disadvantage and the laboratory steps involved in veneer fabrication are technique sensitive and time consuming.[19]

When closing diastemata with a restorative approach, the first dilemma is the mesiodistal enlargement of the teeth on either side of the gap.[20] Careful advance planning is needed to integrate any individual restoration into the whole. When the gap is equal to or less than 1 mm and the teeth are near the ideal proportion, the amount to be added to each tooth will be approximately 0.5 mm. Such a small addition is unlikely to negatively affect tooth proportion. Tooth characterization techniques, such as bringing line angles closer to each other or rounding the distal-incisal corners, can be used on the facial surface to create the illusion of narrower teeth (**Fig. 7**).[20]

If, to maintain proper length to width ratios, teeth need to be lengthened in a diastema closure, it is possible to lengthen the anterior teeth either apically, with periodontal procedures, or incisally with a restorative addition (**Fig. 8**).[1] If the incisal edge position is correct and to be maintained, and there is no periodontal intervention, closing the diastema results in short appearing clinical crowns with disproportional, unattractive teeth. Frequently these patients benefit from a more aggressive restorative approach. It may be necessary to include 4, 6, or more teeth in the restorative plan. The distal surface of the teeth in these cases is reduced with addition to the mesial surface. This approach keeps individual tooth proportion appropriate, while at the same time moves the dental midline to the right position (**Fig. 9**).

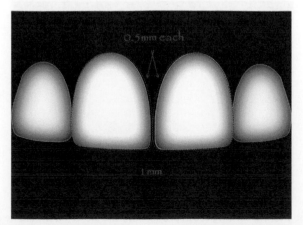

Fig. 7. When the gap is equal to or less than 1 mm, and the teeth are near the ideal proportion, the amount to be added to each tooth will be approximately 0.5 mm.

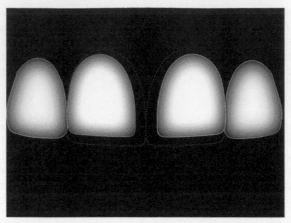

Fig. 8. When teeth exhibit short clinical crowns their lengths should be increased either apically with a periodontal approach, incisally with the restoration or a combination of both modalities.

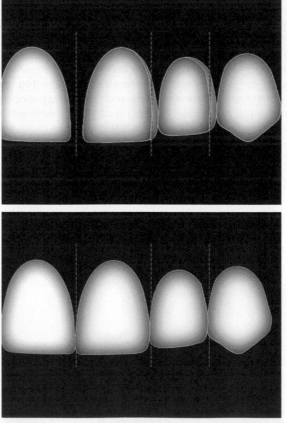

Fig. 9. When not altering existing tooth proportion, the diastema should be closed by using 4 or more teeth. This will permit distalization of the problem by altering both the distal and mesial aspects of the teeth.

Gingival zenith point location must be part of the treatment planning for these cases. If the zenith points are left unchanged from their pretreatment position, they appear to be too far distal. The result is teeth that appear to be mesially tilted. To avoid this outcome, the zenith points have to be relocated with either a periodontal procedure or by recontouring the gingival trough in the provisional restorations (**Fig. 10**).[20]

When performing the preparations for the closure of diastemata, the veneer preparations must be modified. The proximals to be closed are prepared with a slice preparation rather than a wing type preparation. The modification allows the ceramist to create a contact area that transitions to the lingual surface of the tooth without creating a lingual ledge. In addition, depending on the amount of porcelain to be added, the preparation may need to start subgingivally to give the technician sufficient running room to create a natural-appearing clinical crown in the incisogingival direction. In other words, the preparation is modified to avoid overcontouring the emergence profile interproximally. This may also allow pushing and shaping of the gingival papilla. Ideally, the papillae areas will become more pointed and less flat over time (**Fig. 11**).

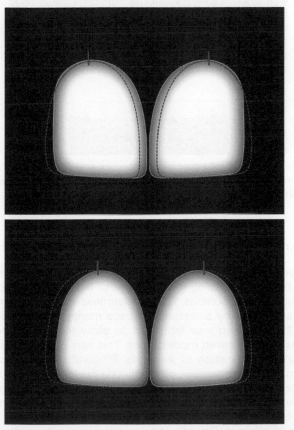

Fig. 10. If the gingival zenith points are left unchanged after the diastema closure, they will be located too far distally and the tooth will appear tilted mesially. This is avoided by relocating the zenith points with either a periodontal procedure or by recontouring the gingival trough in the provisional restorations.

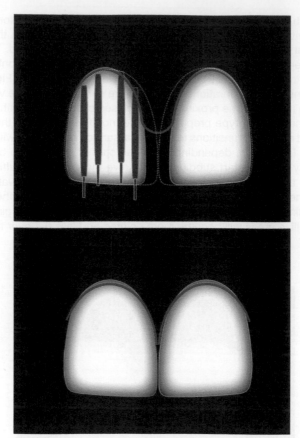

Fig. 11. On the diastema side, the gingival preparation should be located subgingivally so that the emergence profile of the restoration can be slightly over contoured. The resulting gentle push on the papillae will produce the desired triangular shape.

CASE PRESENTATION

The patient presented with a chief compliant of spaces between her teeth. An esthetic evaluation was performed leading to a diagnosis of diastemata associated with peg laterals and poor tooth proportions. It was determined that the patient's complaints could best be addressed by a restorative space management approach to space closure (**Fig. 12**). A wax-up was fabricated to allow the patient, technician, and clinician to visualize the desired modifications. This wax-up indicates the necessary proportion, shape, and position of the teeth. Preparation guides were fabricated from the wax-up. These preparation guides dictate the amount and location of tooth reduction needed during the preparation to achieve the desired goals (**Fig. 13**). Once the guides are tried in the patient's mouth one can see if the case is additive, reductive, or a combination of both. This case was mostly additive, meaning tooth reduction would be minimal (**Fig. 14**). Although not done for this patient, the preparation guides can be used to fabricate a preoperative intraoral mock-up of the final result. In this case, a bis-acrylic mock-up was fabricated intraorally with the help of a transparent silicone impression made from the wax-up. The facial, oral, and tooth

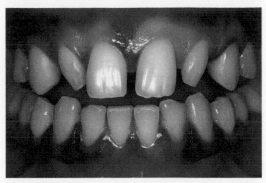

Fig. 12. Genetic factors could lead to tooth malformation, where corrections are needed to restore esthetics and a stable occlusion.

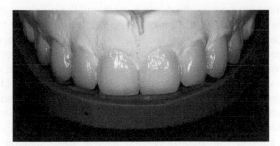

Fig. 13. The diagnostic wax-up serves as a blueprint for the subsequent interdisciplinary treatment and helps the patient visualize the final outcome of the treatment.

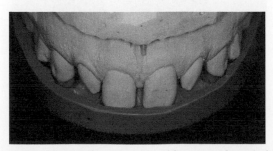

Fig. 14. Preparation guides dictate the amount and location of needed tooth reduction.

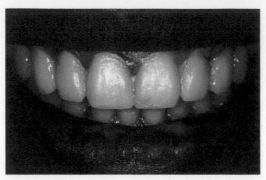

Fig. 15. The mock-up reproducing the diagnostic wax-up serves to reevaluate the patient's function, tooth length, incisal profile and smaller details, and helps the patient visualize the final outcome of the treatment.

proportions, the incisal edge position, the occlusal parameters, speech, and smile were evaluated (**Fig. 15**). At this point, final case acceptance by the patient was obtained.

The preparations were begun with depth cutters and the mock-up in place (**Fig. 16**). The preparation was completed with a diamond bur in such a way that a consistent thickness of porcelain could be developed by the technician. This approach allowed for maximum conservation of enamel and strength of the porcelain veneers. The entire surfaces were then reduced using a round-ended diamond bur at different angles following the convexity of the tooth. The mock-up was cut back until the demarcation lines were removed, indicating that the essential depth was achieved (**Fig. 17**). Once tooth reduction was completed, the preparations were verified by placing the silicone index over the teeth, and sufficient reduction was confirmed. Final impressions were taken and sent to the laboratory with all the specifications needed. In the laboratory, using the guides from the wax-up, the porcelain restorations were initiated (**Fig. 18**). The completed restorations were placed using a 2-step bonding agent (total etch) and light-cured resin cement (**Figs. 19** and **20**).

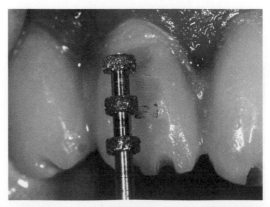

Fig. 16. The depth cutters have a great value in controlling the amount of tooth removed.

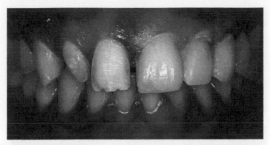

Fig. 17. The entire surface of the mock up was cut back until the demarcation lines were removed.

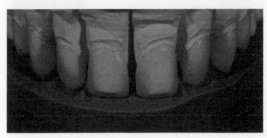

Fig. 18. In the laboratory, the porcelain restorations were initiated using the guides created from wax-up.

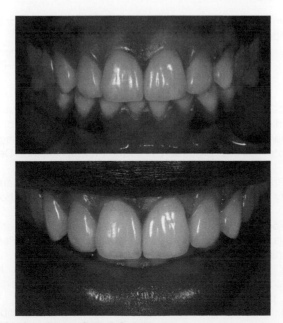

Fig. 19. Final result after the aesthetic rehabilitation.

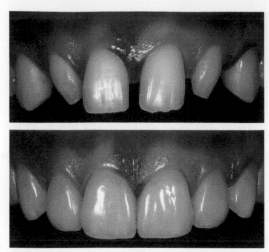

Fig. 20. Maxillary view before and after the case was completed.

SUMMARY

The presence of diastema between teeth is a common feature found in the anterior dentition. Many forms of therapy can be used for diastema closure. A carefully documented diagnosis and treatment plan are essential if the clinician is to apply the most effective approach to address the patient's needs.

ACKNOWLEDGMENTS

The authors thank Dr Stephen Chu and Dr Richard Trushkowsky for their mentoring. Dr Chu also provided the clinical case presented in this article.

REFERENCES

1. Gurel G. Porcelain laminate veneers for diastema closure. In: The science and art of PLV. Ergolding (Germany): Quintessence Publishing; 2003. p. 369–92.
2. Furuse AY, Herkrath FJ, Franco EJ, et al. Multidisciplinary management of anterior diastemata: clinical procedures. Pract Proced Aesthet Dent 2007;19(3): 185–91.
3. Sarver DM. Principles of cosmetic dentistry in orthodontics: part 1. Shape and proportionality of anterior teeth. Am J Orthod Dentofacial Orthop 2004;126(6): 749–53.
4. Chiche G. Proportion, display, and length for successful esthetic planning. In: Cohen M, editor. Interdisciplinary treatment planning. Hanover Park (IL): Quintessence Publishing; 2008. p. 1–47.
5. Sulikowski A. Essential in aesthetics. In: Tarnow D, Chu S, Kim J, editors. Aesthetic restorative dentistry principles and practice. Mahwah (NJ): Montage Media; 2008. p. 27–63.
6. Waldman AB. Smile design for the adolescent patient–interdisciplinary management of anterior tooth size discrepancies. J Calif Dent Assoc 2008;36(5):365–72.

7. De Araujo EM Jr, Fortkamp S, Baratieri LN. Closure of diastema and gingival re-contouring using direct adhesive restorations: a case report. J Esthet Restor Dent 2009;21(4):229–40.
8. Chu S, Tarnow D, Bloom M. Diagnosis, etiology. In: Tarnow D, Chu S, Kim J, editors. Aesthetic restorative dentistry principles and practice. Mahwah (NJ): Montage Media; 2008. p. 1–25.
9. Ward DH. Proportional smile design using the RED proportion. Dent Clin North Am 2001;45(1):143–54.
10. Chu SJ. Range and mean distribution frequency of individual tooth width of the maxillary anterior dentition. Pract Proced Aesthet Dent 2007;19(4):209–15.
11. Gracis S, Chu S. The anterior and posterior determinants of occlusion and their relationship to aesthetic restorative dentistry. In: Tarnow D, Chu S, Kim J, editors. Aesthetic restorative dentistry principles and practice. Mahwah (NJ): Montage Media; 2008. p. 65–97.
12. Dawson P. The envelope of function. In: Functional occlusion: from TMJ to smile design. St. Louis (MO): Mosby Elsevier; 2007. p. 141–7.
13. Chu SJ, Tan J, Stappert CF, et al. Gingival zenith positions and levels of the maxillary anterior dentition. J Esthet Restor Dent 2009;21(2):113–20.
14. Tarnow DP, Magner AW, Fletcher P. The effect of the distance from the contact point to the crest of the bone on the presence or absence of the interproximal dental papilla. J Periodontol 1992;63:995–6.
15. Tarnow D, Cho SC. The interdental papillae. In: Tarnow D, Chu S, Kim J, editors. Aesthetic restorative dentistry principles and practice. Mahwah (NJ): Montage Media; 2008. p. 367–81.
16. Chu S, Tarnow DP, Tan Y, et al. Papilla proportions in the maxillary anterior dentition. Int J Periodontics Restorative Dent 2009;29(4):385–93.
17. Celenza F. Restorative–orthodontic inter-relationships. In: Tarnow D, Chu S, Kim J, editors. Aesthetic restorative dentistry principles and practice. Mahwah (NJ): Montage Media; 2008. p. 427–57.
18. Furuse AY, Franco EJ, Mondelli J. Esthetic and functional restoration for an anterior open occlusal relationship with multiple diastemata: a multidisciplinary approach. J Prosthet Dent 2008;99(2):91–4.
19. Beasley WK, Maskeroni AJ, Moon MG, et al. The orthodontic and restorative treatment of a large diastema: a case report. Gen Dent 2004;52(1):37–41.
20. Gurel G, Chu S, Kim J. Restorative space management. In: Tarnow D, Chu S, Kim J, editors. Aesthetic restorative dentistry principles and practice. Mahwah (NJ): Montage Media; 2008. p. 405–25.

Congenitally Missing Lateral Incisors—A Comparison Between Restorative, Implant, and Orthodontic Approaches

Matthias Krassnig, MD, DDS[a],*, Stefan Fickl, DDS[b]

KEYWORDS

• Tooth agenesis • Hypodontia • Lateral incisors • Orthodontics

Tooth agenesis is one of the most common developmental dental anomalies in humans. Hypodontia describes the absence of 1 to 6 teeth, excluding the third molars. Oligodontia refers to the absence of more than 6 teeth, excluding the third molars, whereas anodontia represents the loss of all the teeth.[1–3] The permanent dentition is more frequently affected than the primary dentition.[1,4,5] There are large discrepancies in the prevalence of dental agenesis between different races.[1,2,4,6–27] Tooth agenesis may appear as part of a recognized genetic syndrome or as a nonsyndrome, familial form, which occurs as an isolated trait.[1,3,28] Recent genetic studies provide information regarding many genes related to both syndrome and nonsyndrome forms of human dental agenesis.

The causes of the most common hypodontia, third molars and incisor-premolar type, are still unknown. An association between PAX9 promoter polymorphisms and hypodontia has been reported,[1,29] so there may be other promoter polymorphisms in genes involved in tooth organogenesis with these types of hypodontia.[1] It is likely that other specific hypodontia genes still exist and will be identified eventually through contributions of molecular genetic research.[1]

Successful and, therefore, satisfying dental treatment is always the goal for both patients and dental practitioners. What does this successful and satisfying treatment

[a] Updent Dentists Vienna, Liechtensteinstrasse 8, 1090 Vienna, Austria
[b] Department of Periodontology, University of Würzburg, Pleicherwall 2, 97070 Würzburg, Germany
* Corresponding author.
E-mail address: mk2923@nyu.edu

Dent Clin N Am 55 (2011) 283–299
doi:10.1016/j.cden.2011.01.004
0011-8532/11/$ – see front matter © 2011 Elsevier Inc. All rights reserved.

mean? It means that a patient's needs are solved in a functional and, more importantly, an esthetic way. This is especially so in the anterior region, where patients react more negatively if the esthetic outcome is not perfect. But the problem dentists are facing is that each patient is an individual, with different parameters according to the smile, smile lines, biotypes according to the gingival tissue and health of the periodontium, habits, and sometimes parafunctional habits. Patients and dentists often face different approaches to achieve the final goal and together they have to find the best way to reach their common goal of satisfaction.

The authors' aim in this article is to introduce and provide examples of different approaches to solve the problem of congenitally missing lateral incisors. Patients with congenitally missing lateral incisors face a problem that is in the middle of the esthetic zone and, therefore, crucial for their biosocial life. Maxillary lateral incisors are congenitally missing in approximately 1% to 2% of the population. They are the third most common congenitally missing teeth, after third molars and lower second premolars. This article discusses the restorative approach, the approach using implants, and the orthodontic approach. Even for the restorative and implant approaches, adjunctive orthodontic treatment is often required to redistribute and/or create the require spaces accordingly. Even if the spaces are closed with orthodontics, restorations may be needed to finish with an esthetic pleasant outcome. In most cases, an interdisciplinary treatment plan has to be worked out and executed. At the end of this article, a fourth approach is touched on, the autotransplantation of teeth. This is a complex interdisciplinary and technique-sensitive approach, but if experienced and skilled specialists are executing it, it can have terrific outcomes not only for congenitally missing lateral incisor cases but also for all sorts of missing teeth in the esthetic zone.

What is the clinical scenario? Imagine that a patient comes into an office and presents with congenitally missing lateral incisors (**Fig. 1**). The patient is then confronted with the option of closing the spaces with canine substitutions or, alternatively, opening up the spaces for an implant or a restoration, such as an acid-etched retained bridge. All options are possible, but the patient is curious as to which one is the most esthetic? Which one is the most esthetic in the long term? What to tell this patient? Are there any established studies that compare the esthetic results of different methods of restoring the missing lateral incisors? Are there certain indications for one type of treatment plan over another

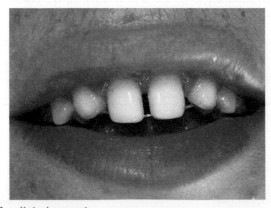

Fig. 1. Example of a clinical scenario.

when considering the malocclusion, smile line, and esthetics of natural teeth? This article aims to provide answers to these questions.

ORTHODONTIC APPROACH

The orthodontic approach is, in the authors' opinion, the most conservative approach and is favorable if a patient meets certain requirements. These requirements are (1) malocclusion and (2) size, shape, and color of the canines.

According to Kokich and Kinzer[30] there are two malocclusions that permit canine substitution (canine repositioning at the site of the lateral incisor). These are an Angle class II malocclusion, with no crowding in the mandibular arch, or an Angle class I malocclusion, with severe crowding in the lower arch where it is necessary to execute extractions. The final occlusion of both variants should end up in an anterior group function in lateral excursive movements.[30–33]

When evaluating the size, shape, and color of the canine carefully, it can be predicted if recontouring alone is enough for an esthetic result or if the orthodontic treatment has to be combined with subsequent restorative treatment. The ideal canine for substitution has similar proportions in width and convexity as the lateral it should replace. Also, the color should be similar to the color of the central incisor. To establish the proper width, either contralateral incisor may be taken as a reference or some proportional calculations can be made. The authors favors Chu's[34] approach with the formula

Central incisor = width in mm = X
Lateral incisor = X − 2 mm
Canine = X − 1 mm

According to this formula by Chu,[34] the canine that substitutes the lateral is approximately 1 mm too wide. That means that 0.5 mm of recontouring mesially and distally would have to be done to get the desired width. The convexity of the lateral incisor is more subtle than the convexity of the canine. Also, the canine normally shows in two planes mesiodistally whereas the lateral incisor has just one. It is also necessary to reshape the lingual surface of the canine to achieve a proper overjet and overbite relation, and the cusp tip of the canine needs enameloplasty as well.

If all this recontouring requires a significant amount of reduction of enamel, problems may occur. One of the problems that can be faced is that a patient experiences dental hypersensitivity, although Zacchrison and Mjör[35] has shown that if all these reductions are performed using diamond instruments with abundant water spray cooling on young teeth, there are no long-term changes in tooth sensitivity. If dentin is exposed, an adjunctive restoration may be necessary.[35–37]

Another problem that occurs is the color of the canine. Usually the canines are one to two shades darker than the central incisor. This problem can get even worse if a lot of reduction has to be performed to flatten a canine with a prominent labial convexity. As the enamel of the canine becomes thinner, the dentin starts to show through the translucent enamel and as a result the tooth appears even darker. One solution for the difference in color is single tooth bleaching, but with thinning the enamel the risk of sensitivity after bleaching increases.[35] Another option is adjunctive restorative treatment.

The bracket placement in canine substitution cases is different. The bracket is not placed with the incisal edge of the canine as a reference but with the gingival margin as the guide. The gingival zeniths of the lateral incisors should be 0.5 to 1 mm lower than the central incisors, so the canine bracket has to be placed accordingly.[35]

To make the final decision if a patient is suitable for the orthodontic approach and to anticipate if additional restorations may be necessary, the authors strongly suggest a carefully executed treatment plan. This treatment plan should include

Full radiographic work-up
Cephalometric analysis
Full esthetic work-up (esthetic evaluation form)
Model analysis for Angle classification and Bolton discrepancies
Model set-up, including the recontoured canine to predict the esthetic and functional result and the amount of reduction (width, labial convexity, incisal, and lingual eminence) necessary to achieve the result.

Advantages
If carefully planned and executed, the orthodontic approach is the most conservative approach (**Figs. 2** and **3**)
Long-term esthetic results
Superior esthetic outcome compared with implants and Maryland bridge according to cohort study
Psychological comfort that the patient has no missing teeth.

Disadvantages
Patient still may need restorative treatment (**Figs. 4** and **5**)
Bleaching or restorations may be necessary if canine appears too dark.

IMPLANT APPROACH

A second option for replacing congenitally missing lateral incisors is to use implant-retained prostheses. In particular, in cases of adjacent teeth devoid of any fillings or color or size issues, placing a single tooth implant may be regarded as the most conservative approach. In addition, various studies have proved that single tooth implants have an excellent long-term result regarding osseointegration and function.[38–42] This is not the case for esthetics, however, because attainment of esthetic rehabilitations with dental implants in the anterior area is currently one of the leading challenges in modern dentistry. The main treatment goals are intact papillae and harmonious gingival contours without any recession of the buccal soft tissue.[38,43,44] The height of the peri-implant papillae for single tooth implants is not determined by the peri-implant bone level but rather the bone level of the adjacent teeth.[38,45,46] Therefore, an optimal 3-D implant placement should include at least 1.5 mm of distance between the implant and the adjoining teeth (**Fig. 6**). Additionally, as in most cases, soft and hard tissue structure is missing; augmentative procedures

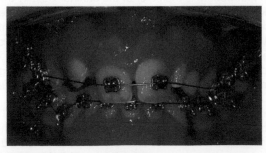

Fig. 2. Orthodontic approach during treatment.

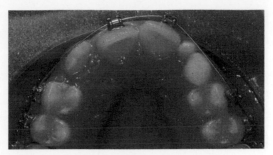

Fig. 3. Orthodontic approach during treatment.

have to be performed at the time of implant placement or at the time of abutment connection.

Several criteria have to be considered before placing a single tooth implant in adolescents:

1. Time of implant placement
2. Development of a proper implant site
3. Space needed coronally
4. Space needed apically
5. Height of gingiva
6. Retention of space needed before implant placement.

Time of Implant Placement

It is of major importance when considering implant-retained prostheses to evaluate if the skeletal growth of a patient is still active. Studies have demonstrated that cranio-facial growth continues on average until age 17 for women and 21 for men.[35,38,47] A more precise estimation of the individual growth pattern of an implant patient can be performed, however, with hand-wrist radiographs. A second option is to use the cervical vertebral maturation developed by Baccetti and colleagues,[48] who produced diagrammatic drawings and descriptions of 6 stages of cervical vertebral maturation. They evaluated the cervical maturation by the changes in the concavity of the lower border, height, and shape of the vertebral body. When considering implant placement, deep concavities have to be observed on the second, third, and fourth cervical verte-brae, and the vertebral bodies display a greater vertical than horizontal dimension (completion phase). This information can be retrieved from a lateral cephalometric radiograph, which is routinely obtained by an orthodontist. The most precise instru-ment to assess the completion of the facial growth is superimpositions of lateral ceph-alometric radiographs.[45,47] These radiographs should be obtained 6 months to 1 year

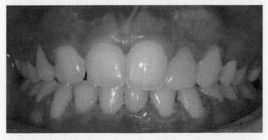

Fig. 4. Patient after orthodontic treatment and additional restoration.

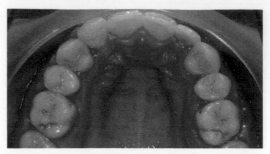

Fig. 5. Patient after orthodontic treatment and additional restoration.

apart. The facial growth can be regarded as complete if the distance from nasion to menton is stable within 1 year.

Development of a Proper Implant Site

To achieve a predictable and esthetically satisfying implant outcome, it is crucial to have a properly developed implant site (**Fig. 7**). The buccolingual dimension of the alveolar ridge has to be wide enough to allow a surgeon to place the implant in a correct 3-D position.

If the buccolingual dimension is insufficient, a bone graft may be necessary. An ideal method to develop a proper width of the alveolar ridge can be achieved if the canine erupts next to the central incisor. The buccolingual width of the canine creates a sufficient width of the ridge when erupting. After eruption, the canine can be distalized orthodontically and, therefore, establish a proper buccopalatal width of the alveolar ridge. Studies have demonstrated that if an implant site is developed with this kind of orthodontic guided tooth movement, the buccopalatal width remains stable. Distalizing may need to be done with bodily movement to develop adequate space between the roots. If a panoramic radiograph reveals that the permanent canine is apical to the primary canine, the extraction of the primary lateral incisor may be considered to guide the eruption of the permanent canine toward the central incisor.[38,49–51] This (as explained previously) is favorable for developing a proper implant site. Otherwise, it may not be possible to guide the eruption of the canine near the central incisor, the osseous ridge will not fully develop, and the buccopalatal width will be insufficient for a proper implant placement. In these cases, it is necessary to perform a bone graft before or at the time of implant placement to achieve a sufficient dimension of the alveolar ridge.

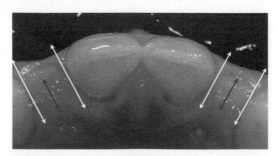

Fig. 6. Space management for implant placement.

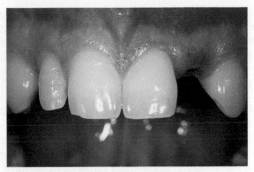

Fig. 7. Implant placed in position #10.

Space Needed Coronally

The assessment of the space available mesiodistally is crucial to evaluate the diameter of the implant. In unilateral congenitally missing lateral incisor cases, the contralateral lateral incisor may be used for assessing the proper mesiodistal space needed. In cases of peg-shaped contralateral lateral incisors or when both lateral incisors are congenitally missing, other tools have to be used. One of these tools may be a formula initiated by Chu[34]:

Central incisor = X
Lateral incisor = X − 2 mm
Canine = X − 1 mm

Another way to estimate the correct dimension of the lateral incisiors is to use the Bolton analysis. By this means, the mesiodistal widths of the arches can be compared to achieve an ideal occlusal relationship. It is an easy and efficient way to mathematically calculate the proper width of the missing lateral incisor. The best tool, however, for assessing the ideal width of the missing lateral incisor is a diagnostic wax-up. In particular, for multidisciplinary cases, it facilitates an overview for both the orthodontist and the restorative dentist. Another advantage is the visualization for patients so that the final outcome can be imagined and patients can provide input into alterations of the esthetic outcome.

Attention has to be given to the minimal mesiodistal width that is needed for the implant per se. A minimum of 5.5 mm is required. There should be at least 1 mm distance between the implant and the adjacent teeth; otherwise, the interproximal bone could be jeopardized, and the space for the papilla between the implant crown and adjacent teeth is constricted and appears much shorter than the papillae on the contralateral side.[39] A disagreeable esthetic outcome would be the result.

Space Needed Apically

Careful attention has to be paid to the distance of the apical roots between central incisor and canine. A minimum of 5 mm is required generally to provide sufficient space for a 3.5-mm implant. This space has to be provided by an orthodontist, who controls the mesiodistal root angulation when creating space for an implant. During this process of creating space, the mesiodistal space coronally is achieved earlier due to a so-called tipping movement, followed by a change of the mesiodistal angulation of the roots. It is crucial not to rely on the appearance of the mesiodistal distance of the coronal aspect, which is achieved earlier than the proper mesiodistal distance of the roots. Not paying attention to this aspect leads to too early removal of the ortho-dontic appliances and, therefore, insufficient space between the roots. To prevent this mistake, radiographs of this particular area should be made to make sure that suffi-cient interradicular space is created before removal of orthodontic appliances.

Height of Gingival Margins

In most implant systems, the distance between the head of the implant and the future gingival margin has to be 4 mm (**Figs. 8** and **9**). In adolescents, many times the alveolar bone is at the level of the cementoenamel junction of the adjacent teeth. In compar-ison, in adults, the alveolar bone is 2 mm apical to the cementoenamel junction. Thus it is sometimes necessary in adolescent patients to perform gingival surgeries, including or excluding bone removal, before the implant placement can be done.

Another aspect of the gingival papillae is that when teeth are moved in adults during space opening, the papilla remains stationary and the adjacent sulci are averted.[38] The nonkeratinized gingiva appears red at first and keratinizes over time; just the papilla itself does not move. The good news is that most patients are treated during adolescence; thus, this phenomenon of a stationary papilla does not occur with them. Therefore, there are no esthetic issues with the papillae adjacent to the lateral incisor implant in adolescents.

Retention of Space Needed Before Implant Placement

As discussed previously, as a general guide, implants can be placed in women at approximately age 17 and in men at approximately age 21. At these ages, craniofacial growth is generally completed. Treatment of these patients should start before this age because development of the alveolar ridge has to be achieved and coronal space and interradicular space has to be created. That leads to a period of time when space maintenance may have to be provided for a patient, if craniofacial growth is not yet completed. The temporization and stabilization depends on the waiting time until the implant may be placed. If patients are ready for implant placement in a couple of months, a removable retainer, such as a Hawley retainer or an Essix retainer with a built-in prosthetic tooth, can be used. If patients have to wait 1 or 2 years before completion of growth is achieved, a temporary resin-bonded bridge is the more favor-able option.

Advantages of implant approach
No adjacent teeth have to be prepared (see **Figs. 7–9; Fig. 10**)
Successful osseointegration of implants.

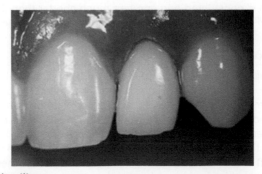

Fig. 8. Soft tissue detailing.

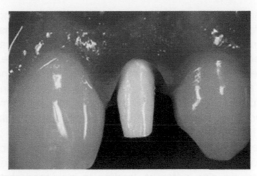

Fig. 9. Nicely formed soft tissue.

Disadvantages of implant approach
>   Esthetic outcome may be worse than orthodontic approach and/or prosthetic
>   approach (long term)
>   Needs perfect team play between orthodontist, oral surgeon, and prosthodon-
>   tist or result could be compromised
>   Apical migration of gingival and bone if traditional implants are used—additional
>   need of grafting overtime to obtain esthetic results.

RESTORATIVE APPROACH

Another approach to congenitally missing lateral incisors is the restorative approach.
The restorative approach may be categorized as (1) resin-bonded bridge, (2) conventional bridge, and (3) cantilever bridge.

Resin-Bonded Bridge

Of the possibilities for a restorative approach, the resin-bonded bridge is the most
conservative option. The reason is that contrary to the conventional bridge and the
cantilever bridge, it leaves the adjacent teeth relatively untouched. The resin-
bonded bridge relies on adhesion alone; no pins or retention grooves are necessary.
The literature gives a wide variation of failure rates, from 54% over 11 months to 10%
over 10 years.[45–47,49,50]

Ideally, resin-bonded bridges should be considered if an overbite is shallow or just
deep enough to provide anterior guidance to disclude the posterior teeth. The reason

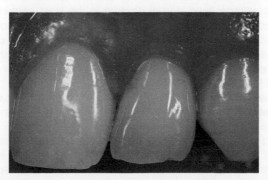

Fig. 10. Final result.

is that a shallow overbite leaves a maximum surface area for bonding without the need for too much preparation of the adjacent teeth. Another advantage is a decrease in the amount of lateral force in the abutment teeth. In deep overbite situations, the amount of forces is increased, so the stress increases on the bond interface, and that leads to a higher failure rate in deep bite situations.[45,51] Also, the interincisal angle found between the upper and lower incisors plays a role. A higher interincisal angle corresponds with more upright upper and lower incisors, leading to more shear forces, which can withstand 40% more load before failure compared with the same object loaded with tensile forces.[45]

The abutment teeth of resin-bonded bridges should not be mobile. The reason is that if the mobility of the two abutment teeth is different from each other, the force vectors when loaded are also different, leading to increased stress in comparison with normal abutment teeth. In addition, parafunction, such as bruxism, makes resin-bonded bridges less favorable.

Esthetically, the thickness and translucency of resin-bonded bridges can be challenging when the wings are made of metal. This can lead sometimes to a grayish appearance of the abutment teeth and is a contraindication. A solution for avoiding this grayish appearance can be the so-called encore bridge. Instead of metal wings, this kind of resin-bonded bridge incorporates laboratory-processed composite resin with fiber reinforcement in the form of a lingual framework with a ceramic veneer bonded to the facial of the pontic. Unlike metal, the fiber-reinforced resin body framework readily bonds to enamel and dentin and has strength and flexibility to resist fracture or debonding, even if the abutment teeth are slightly mobile. Because of the tooth-colored material of the framework, the problem of discoloration and grayish appearance of the enamel caused by metal show-through is eliminated. Although different preparation designs exist for the encore bridge, it seems that the one that incorporates as much of the lingual surface as possible (depth approximately 1 mm) and has a horizontal central groove for strength, a proximal box design for increased thickness, and fiber concentration in the connector sides has the best long-term results.[51]

The ideal candidate for a resin-bonded bridge has

Shallow overbite
Nonmobile abutment teeth
Moderate thickness of abutment teeth
Translucency mainly in the incisal third of the abutment teeth.[45]

Conventional Full-Coverage Fixed Partial Denture

Conventional full-coverage fixed partial denture is the least conservative approach regarding the adjacent teeth (**Figs. 11–15**). Therefore, it should not be a treatment option in adolescent, virgin teeth without any fillings, discolorations, or issues in shape and size. It is a treatment option that can be considered if there is already an existing restoration on the abutment teeth, if there are discolorations, and/or if shape and size have to be altered (see **Figs. 11–13**).

If orthodontic therapy is required before the full-coverage fixed partial denture, it can help significantly in positioning the teeth in an ideal inclination and angulations for the abutment teeth, so that overpreparation can be avoided.

When evaluating a patient's teeth from a frontal perspective, the long axis of the central incisor and the canine should be parallel. The same long axis occurs when looking at a patient's central incisor and canine from a lateral perspective. The long axis should be parallel as well for a proper tooth preparation. These teeth are often

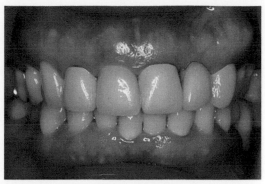

Fig. 11. Old restoration with bridge #9–11 to replace #10.

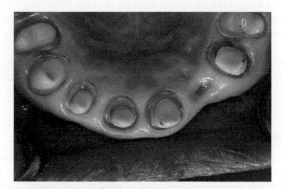

Fig. 12. View at missing #10 with deficient alveolar ridge.

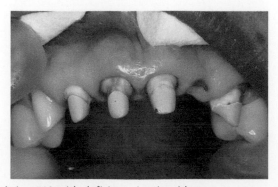

Fig. 13. View at missing #10 with deficient alveolar ridge.

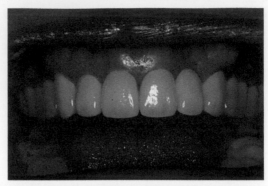

Fig. 14. New restoration with new bridge to replace #10.

collapsed or tipped into the edentulous space of the missing lateral incisor, and an orthodontist is able to recreate these ideal parallel inclinations and make the preparation of the abutment teeth simple for a prosthodontist. The orthodontist should be able to know the limits of the envelope of the alveolar bone in order to provide proper feedback to the prosthodontist when not able to achieve an ideal axial inclination. In doing so, the dental team can consider changing the treatment plan to better suit a particular patient.

Finishing orthodontic treatment leaving the patient with an increased overjet or open bite can be favourable in combined orthodontic-restorative cases as this leaves more space for the prosthodontist allowing for more minimally invasive preparations of abutment teeth.[45]

Cantilever Fixed Partial Denture

The cantilever fixed partial denture uses the canine as an abutment tooth. This kind of restoration can be executed either as a full-coverage preparation or more conservatively as a partial cover denture, which needs pins for additional retention and resistance. The placements of pins require extra care and caution in adolescents due to a large pulpal chamber.

Careful attention has to be paid to the management of the occlusion of the pontic tooth.[45,52,53] The contacts in laterotrusion movements have to be removed from the pontic; otherwise, there is high risk of fracture, loosening the restoration and migration of the canine.[45]

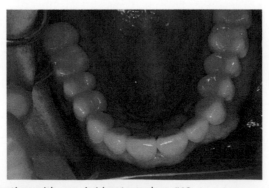

Fig. 15. New restoration with new bridge to replace #10.

Important in the prosthodontic planning and actual treatment of children and adolescents is the adaption to these growing individuals, meaning that the growth potential has to be respected; therefore, it is not acceptable to treat growing individuals with any kind of final fixed partial dentures. Solutions, until growth has finally ceased, are interim prostheses, such as resin-bonded fixed partial dentures with only one abutment tooth and 3-D self-adjusting fixed partial dentures.[54]

Advantages of restorative approach
1. Occlusal and esthetic adjustments can be built in the restoration (full-coverage fixed partial dentures)
2. Fast approach if no orthodontic treatment needed.

Disadvantages of restorative approach
1. Least conservative approach
2. Additional orthodontic treatment may be needed
3. Has to be changed over lifetime; additional preparation may be necessary.

THE AUTOTRANSPLANTATION APPROACH

An entirely different, but, if executed carefully and in a sophisticated manner, highly satisfactorily approach is the autotransplantation of premolars to the site of missing incisors. This approach was developed 45 years ago by Slagsvold and Bjercke.[55,56] The optimal time for the autotransplantation of premolars to the maxillary incisor area is when the development of the roots of the premolars has reached two-thirds to three-fourths of the final root length.[55–57] If the timing is right, which means patients are approximately 9 to 12 years of age, the periodontal healing is better than 90%.[55,57] Root growth continues after the autotransplantation and the teeth maintain their capacity for functional adaption; endodontic treatment is most of the time not necessary after treatment. Next to timing, the surgical technique for tooth transplant is of great importance for the success of the treatment, which means that any damage of the periodontal ligament has to be avoided; otherwise, alkalosis may occur.[55]

The long-term results for autotransplantation are impressive. Czochrowska and colleagues[58,59] found, in their long-term studies, including 33 transplanted premolars with a mean of 26.4 years, a survival rate of 90%.

Additional orthodontic treatment after autotransplantation is possible, because a normal periodontal ligament is established. Waiting 3 to 4 months is recommended before any orthodontic treatment is started.[55] The premolars are usually reshaped and build up with composite in the beginning; later on, when an ideal result is achieved, the composites can be replaced with porcelain veneers.

Advantages of autotransplantation approach
Biologic approach
Creates alveolar bone
Periodontal membrane
Adjustable alveolar bone
Periodontal membrane after surgery with orthodontics
Normal interdental papilla
Good long-term results.

Disadvantages of autotransplantation approach
Experienced surgeon necessary
Very technique sensitive
Age limitation, 9–12.

SUMMARY

The concern for esthetics is an ever-growing demand and goal in today's dental treatment plans provided to patients. In the past, function, biology, and structure were more important; esthetics had to follow. Today, it should be the goal to start with the best esthetic outcome in mind and then work out the treatment plan according to it. That does not mean that function, biology, and structure are less important than before; it just means that the esthetic goal should be set first, not at the end of the treatment. As Dawson said, "if know where you are, and if you know where you are (esthetically) going, getting there is easy."

As discussed previously, many instances need a team play of several specialties to reach the optimal esthetic result for individuals. It is important that every member of the team is exactly aware of what he or she has to do; otherwise, the result may become compromised or even disastrous. Such complications may be avoided by systematically designing a multidisciplinary treatment plan in which individual responsibilities are detailed in chronologic order, so that everybody has a clear picture of what to do and what the team players have to do.

Specifically, for missing congenitally lateral incisors there are several treatment options, which all can lead to a good result if patients are properly selected for an ideal treatment. Canine substitution can be a good treatment solution, if certain criteria are met. Nevertheless, team play with a restorative dentist is often required to reach an optimal esthetic outcome. Also, the restorative option can be used to meet a patient's high esthetic demands, if used in the right situation; hence, requiring an interdisciplinary treatment approach is often necessary to get the best result. Implants are probably the most favorable treatment alternative for many dentists for replacing missing anterior teeth. The implant approach in the anterior region is a delicate situation, which can be challenging esthetically, especially in the long term. In this scenario, it is necessary to work as a team to have ideal conditions before and after implant placement. Autotransplantation can be a good alternative in growing patients. It is not suitable for nongrowing adults. As in all the other treatment options, an interdisciplinary approach between oral surgeon, periodontist, orthodontist, and restorative dentist is crucial. This may be the most important take-home message in today's world: with the high demand for esthetics, it is not possible for a dentist who tries to work alone to achieve an optimal esthetic result, especially in challenging cases. Furthermore, it is imperative to have the best people in every specialty working together to satisfy patients' esthetic needs. More importantly, there should not be a scenario where several specialists are working on a case but one where all these specialists are working together on a case. This ideal equilibrium between all the different specialists defines the interdisciplinary team approach, which will lead to the best esthetic outcome possible.

ACKNOWLEDGMENTS

We want to thank Dr Walter Wadsak and Associates for providing Figs. 1–5 and 11–15 for the restorative and orthodontic parts of this article. Furthermore, we would like to thank Dr Steven David for editing this article and Dr Richard Trushkowsky for organizing and supporting the writing of this article.

REFERENCES

1. Shimizu T, Maeda T. Prevalence and genetic basis of tooth agenesis. Jpn Dent Sci Rev 2009;45:52–8.

2. Goya HA, Tanaka S, Maeda T, et al. An orthopantomographic study of hypodontia in permanent teeth of Japanese pediatric patients. J Oral Sci 2008;50:143–50.
3. Stockton DW, Das P, Goldenberg M, et al. Mutation of PAX9 is associated with oligodontia. Nat Genet 2000;24:18–9.
4. Terasaki T, Shiota K. Congenital absence of teeth. Nihon Koku Kagakkai Zasshi 1954;3:88–93 [in Japanese].
5. Ogita S, Ogita M, Yamamoto T, et al. The appearance of supernumerary teeth and congenitally missing teeth in Japanese pediatric patients. Aichi Gakuin Daigaku Shigakkai Shi 1995;33:19–27 [in Japanese].
6. Okamoto O, Mori O, Morimoto M, et al. A statistical and genetic study related to congenital missing teeth. Shikwa Gakuho 1951;5:39–46 [in Japanese].
7. Tsutsui H, Yoshida Y. Clinical statistical study on supernumerary teeth and congenital absence of teeth. Kokubyo Gakkai Zasshi 1955;22:44–8 [in Japanese].
8. Niswander JD, Sujaku C. Congenital anomalies of teeth in Japanese children. Am J Phys Anthropol 1963;21:569–74.
9. Nakahara M, Okada S, Tani H, et al. A survey of congenitally missing permanent teeth in Hokkaido. Koku Eisei Gakkai Zasshi 1977;27:21–3 [in Japanese].
10. Ishizuka K, Sasaki T, Imai R, et al. Anomalies of teeth which affects the orthodontic treatment. Nichidai Shigaku 1988;62:584–95 [in Japanese].
11. Yanagida I, Mori S. Statistical studies on numerical anomalies of teeth in children using orthopantomograms: congenital hypodontia. Osaka Daigaku Shigaku Zasshi 1990;35:580–93 [in Japanese].
12. Hirukawa K, Iwata R, Kurosawa M, et al. Statistical investigation about the prevalence of congenitally missing permanent teeth. Nippon Kyosei Shika Gakkai Zasshi 1999;58:49–56 [in Japanese].
13. Endo T, Ozoe R, Kubota M, et al. A survey of hypodontia in Japanese orthodontic patients. Am J Orthod Dentofacial Orthop 2006;129:29–35.
14. Davis PJ. Hypodontia and hyperdontia of permanent teeth in Hong Kong schoolchildren. Community Dent Oral Epidemiol 1987;15:218–20.
15. Nik-Hussein NN. Hypodontia in the permanent dentition: a study of its prevalence in Malaysian children. Aust Orthod J 1989;11:93–5.
16. Albashaireh ZS, Khader YS. The prevalence and pattern of hypodontia of the permanent teeth and crown size and shape deformity affecting upper lateral incisors in a sample of Jordanian dental patients. Community Dent Health 2006;23:239–43.
17. Altug-Atac AT, Erdem D. Prevalence and distribution of dental anomalies in orthodontic patients. Am J Orthod Dentofacial Orthop 2007;131:510–4.
18. Bergström K. An orthopantomographic study of hypodontia, supernumeraries and other anomalies in school children between the ages of 8–9 years. An epidemiological study. Swed Dent J 1977;1:145–57.
19. Rolling S. Hypodontia of permanent teeth in Danish schoolchildren. Scand J Dent Res 1980;88:365–9.
20. Aasheim B, Ogaard B. Hypodontia in 9-year-old Norwegians related to need of orthodontic treatment. Scand J Dent Res 1993;101:257–60.
21. Nordgarden H, Jensen JL, Storhaug K. Reported prevalence of congenitally missing teeth in two Norwegian counties. Community Dent Health 2002;19:258–61.
22. O'Dowling IB, McNamara TG. Congenital absence of permanent teeth among Irish school-children. J Ir Dent Assoc 1990;36:136–8.
23. Rose JS. A survey of congenitally missing teeth, excluding third molars, in 6000 orthodontic patients. Dent Pract Dent Rec 1966;17:107–14.

24. Magnússon TE. Prevalence of hypodontia and malformations of permanent teeth in Iceland. Community Dent Oral Epidemiol 1977;5:173–8.

25. Thompson GW, Popovich F. Probability of congenitally missing teeth: results in 1,191 children in the Burlington Growth centre in Toronto. Community Dent Oral Epidemiol 1974;2:26–32.

26. Byrd ED. Incidence of supernumerary and congenitally missing teeth. J Dent Child 1943;10:84–6.

27. Muller TP, Hill IN, Petersen AC, et al. A survey of congenitally missing permanent teeth. J Am Dent Assoc 1970;81:101–7.

28. Frazier-Bowers SA, Guo DC, Cavender A, et al. A novel mutation in human PAX9 causes molar oligodontia. J Dent Res 2002;81:129–33.

29. Peres RC, Scarel-Caminaga RM, do Espírito Santo AR, et al. Association between PAX-9 promoter polymorphisms and hypodontia in humans. Arch Oral Biol 2005; 50:861–71.

30. Kokich VG, Kinzer GA. Managing congenitally missing lateral incisors, part I: Canine substitution. J Esthet Restor Dent 2005;17:1–6.

31. Zachrisson BU. Improving orthodontic results in cases with maxillary incisors missing. Am J Orthod 1978;73:274–89.

32. Tuverson DL. Orthodontic treatment using canines in place of missing maxillary lateral incisors. Am J Orthod 1970;58:109–27.

33. Senty EL. The maxillary cuspid and missing lateral incisors: esthetics and occlusion. Angle Orthod 1976;46:365–71.

34. Chu SJ. Range and mean distribution frequency of individual tooth width of maxillary anterior dentition. Pract Proced Aesthet Dent 2007;19:209–15.

35. Zachrisson BU, Mjör IA. Remodeling of teeth by grinding. Am J Orthod 1975;68: 545–53.

36. Sabri R. Management of missing lateral incisors. J Am Dent Assoc 1999;130: 80–4.

37. Thordarson A, Zachrisson BU, Mjor IA. Remodeling of canines to the shape of lateral incisors by grinding: a long-term clinical and radiographic evaluation. Am J Orthod Dentofacial Orthop 1991;100:123–32.

38. Kinzer GA, Kokich VG. Managing congenitally missing lateral incisors. Part III: single-tooth implants. J Esthet Restor Dent 2005;17:202–10.

39. Wenig D, Jacobsen Z, Tarnow D, et al. A prospective multicenter clinical trial of 3i machined-surface implants: results after 6 years of follow-up. Int J Oral Maxillofac Implants 2003;18:417–23.

40. Davarpanah M, Martinez H, Etienne D, et al. A prospective multicenter evaluation of 1,583 3i implants. 1 to 5-year data. Int J Oral Maxillofac Implants 2002;17: 820–8.

41. Romeo E, Chiapasco M, Ghisolfi M, et al. Long term clinical effectiveness of oral implants in the treatment of partial edentulism. Seven year life table analysis of a prospective study with ITI dental implants systems used for single tooth restorations. Clin Oral Implants Res 2002;13(2):133–43.

42. Noack N, Willer J, Hoffmann J. Long-term results after placement of dental implants: longitudinal study of 1,964 implants over 16 years. Int J Oral Maxillofac Implants 1999;14:748–55.

43. McNeill RW, Joondeph DR. Congenitally absent maxillary lateral incisors: treatment planning considerations. Angle Orthod 1973;43:24–9.

44. Nordquist GG, McNeil RW. Orthodontic vs. restorative treatment of the congenitally absent lateral incisor-long term periodontal and occlusal evaluation. J Periodontol 1975;46:139–43.

45. Spear F, Mathews D, Kokich VG. Interdisciplinary management of single tooth implants. Semin Orthod 1997;3:45–72.
46. Saadun AP, LeGall M, Touati B. Current trends in implantology: part II-treatment planning in tissue regeneration. Pract Periodontics Aesthet Dent 2004;16:707–14.
47. Fudalej P, Kokich VG, Leroux B. Determining the cessation of vertical growth of the craniofacial structures to facilitate placement of single-tooth implants. Am J Orthod Dentofacial Orthop 2007;131(Suppl 4):S59–67.
48. Baccetti T, Franchi L, McNamara JA. The Cervical Maturation (CVM) method for the assessment of optimal treatment timing in dentofacial orthopedics. Semin Orthod 2005;11(3):119–29.
49. Kokich VG. Maxillary lateral incisor implants:planning with the aid of orthodontics. Int J Oral Maxillofac Surg 2004;62:48–56.
50. Ostler MS, Kokich VG. Alveolar ridge changes in patients congenitally missing mandibular second premolars. J Prosthet Dent 1994;71:144–9.
51. Biggerstaff RH. The orthodontic management of congenitally absent maxillary lateral incisors and second premolars: a case report. Am J Orthod Dentofacial Orthop 1992;102:537–45.
52. Kelly JR, Tesk JA, Sorensen JA. Failure of all-ceramic fixed partial dentures in vitro and in vivo: analysis and modeling. J Dent Res 1995;74:1253–8.
53. Oh WS, Anusavice KJ. Effect of connector design on the fracture resistance of all-ceramic fixed partial dentures. J Prosthet Dent 2002;87:536–42.
54. Burghard P. Optimizing esthetics for implant rehabilitation in maxillary lateral incisors aplasia: multidisciplinary considerations and 7 years follow-up case report. Stomatologie 2009;106(8):157–63.
55. Zachrisson B, Stenvik A, Haanaes H. Management of missing maxillary anterior teeth with emphasis on autotransplantation. Am J Orthod Dentofacial Orthop 2004;126:284–8.
56. Slagsvold O, Bjercke B. Applicability of autotransplantation in cases of missing upper anterior teeth. Am J Orthod 1978;74:410–21.
57. Kristerson L. Autotransplantation of human premolars. A clinical and radiographic study of 100 teeth. Int J Oral Surg 1985;14:200–13.
58. Zachrisson B. Planning esthetic treatment after avulsion of maxillary incisors. J Am Dent Assoc 2008;139(11):1484–90.
59. Czochrowska EM, Stenvik A, Bjercke B, et al. Outcome of tooth transplantation: survival and success rates 17–41 years post-treatment. Am J Orthod Dentofacial Orthop 2002;121(2):110–9.

Dental Crowding: The Restorative Approach

Luis Brea, DDS*, Anabella Oquendo, DDS, Steven David, DMD

KEYWORDS

- Crowding • Insufficient space • Dentoalveolar discrepancies
- Orthodontic

Dental crowding can be simply defined as the overlap of teeth caused by insufficient space within the dental arch.[1] This article addresses the apparent versus real correction of crowding within the esthetic zone. Crowding of anterior teeth usually has both a mesiodistal and buccolingual component. Drifting, aberrant eruption patterns, habits, tooth size discrepancies, space loss caused by early loss of deciduous teeth, and interproximal caries promoting migration are the typical contributing factors to the occurrence of crowding.[1,2] Because the gingival alveolar complex conforms to the shape and position of the teeth, treatment planning for the correction of anterior crowding must include treatment considerations for the associated gingival discrepancies.[3] As is the case for diastemata, in which excess intra-arch space exists, the treatment of anterior crowding presents the challenge of not only satisfying the patient's desire to correct the esthetic deformity but also to provide the patient with a stable and functional result.[4,5] This article considers the criteria for choosing a totally restorative, or so-called diamond (as in diamond bur) orthodontic, approach versus the need for a traditional orthodontic approach. Finding a conservative and biologically sound treatment plan in every clinical situation is the ideal goal. As is also true for diastemata, the participation of several dental disciplines is frequently required to accomplish the goal of esthetic correction of the crowded dentition.[3] A clear understanding of the roles of the various disciplines in developing and executing the treatment plan is essential.[6] Considerations include the variations and classification of dental crowding from the restorative perspective, the importance of orthodontic therapy, and why orthodontics may be appropriate in every treatment plan.[3,6]

CLASSIFICATION OF DENTAL CROWDING

The degree of teeth misalignment directly influences the treatment options,[3] and at times it can be difficult to define the difference between, mild, moderate, and severe

Department of Cariology and Comprehensive Care, New York University College of Dentistry, New York, NY, USA
* Corresponding author. 2 Cottontail Road, Norwalk, CT 06854.
E-mail address: Lbrea16@gmail.com

Dent Clin N Am 55 (2011) 301–310
doi:10.1016/j.cden.2011.01.010
0011-8532/11/$ – see front matter © 2011 Published by Elsevier Inc.

dental.theclinics.com

levels of dental crowding.[5] There are 2 components to consider in every case of crowding: the mesiodistal overlap and the buccolingual overlap. The amount of overlap can be measured in millimeters, classifying dental crowding according to its severity.[3] Chu's classification makes dental crowding variants less subjective and is therefore a valuable diagnostic tool in the process of treatment planning (**Fig. 1**).[3,5] In the ideal clinical situation, minor to moderate mesiodistal and buccolingual discrepancies can be corrected by restorative means. The management of severe discrepancies solely by restorative care is contraindicated by required tooth mutilation and possibly extensive support compromising periodontal surgery.[3] The degree of vertical discrepancy is another component of crowding to be considered (**Fig. 2**).[7] Lack of proper centric stops may result in supraeruption of the teeth.[7] The esthetically aberrant overerupted tooth, often with an aberrant alveolar gingival complex, is best treated with orthodontic intrusion. Supraeruption presents a restorative challenge because it can lead to overpreparation and the necessity for periodontal intervention.[7-9] Any treatment modality for the crowded dentition should be designed to achieve form and function with minimal invasive dentistry. Esthetics, periodontal health and architecture, structural stability, and occlusion require equally careful attention. The patient's long-term interests are best served by an approach that considers all these elements.[3-5]

THE ROLL OF ORTHODONTICS

The number of adult patients seeking treatment to make an improvement in the appearance of their teeth is increasing, and so are the treatment options. Because of the diversity of dental histories, personal objectives, and treatment demands such as invisible appliances and short treatment times, the orthodontist is often challenged by the adult population.[10] Objectives can often be related to occupational demands and an aversion to unusual appearance during the treatment phase.[3]

MESIO-DISTAL CLASSIFICATION	AMOUNT OF OVERLAP M-D	
0	No Overlap	
1	1mm or less	
2	>1mm to 2mm	
3	>2mm to 3mm	
4	>3mm	
BUCCO-LINGUAL CLASSIFICATION	**AMOUNT OF OVERLAP B-L**	
0	No Overlap	
1	1mm or less	
2	>1mm to 2mm	
3	>2mm to 3mm	
4	>3mm	

Fig. 1. Stephen Chu's classification table.

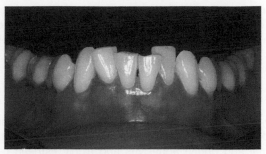

Fig. 2. The extrusion of tooth 23; without orthodontics the restorative approach will result in tooth mutilation and unneeded periodontal surgery.

The incorporation of newer techniques and materials, such as clear and spring-removable aligners, has increased patient acceptance.[3] These removable devices are entirely compliance dependent and may not be suitable in all clinical situations.[11] Nevertheless, their use has increased. In more demanding cases, in which intrusion, extrusion, and torquing movements are necessary, the use of conventional fixed orthodontics is usually recommended.[11] The availability of clear brackets, ceramic brackets, and lingual orthodontics for fixed appliances has also contributed to patient acceptance.[10]

The use of orthodontic tooth movement to correct misalignment has the added benefit of affecting the alveolar-periodontal complex by remodeling the interproximal and midfacial soft tissues. Surgical intervention is thereby obviated (**Fig. 3**).[6] When using orthodontics to influence a crowded dentition, posttreatment retention is indispensable to ensure the long-term stability of the final result. The basic rule is that any tooth that is moved will require retention. Without retention there will be some relapse. Each tooth will move toward its original position.[3,11] In adults, if tissue remodeling is time consuming, the importance of planning adequate retention cannot be overstated.[8,11] It is the appearance of the natural crowns that is disturbing in the crowded dentition. However, the underlying problem is the improper spread of the roots. Posttreatment relapse is the consequence of treatment of the crowns without also addressing the root issues.[12] From the perspective of case management and end result, orthodontic repositioning before restoration offers functional and esthetic

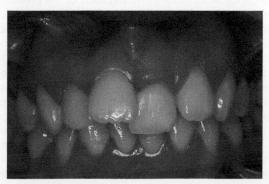

Fig. 3. Interproximal and midfacial gingival architecture discrepancies teeth 8, 9, and 10. Remodeling requires the aid of orthodontics.

advantages. In planning correction of the crowded dentition, the dentist should make the extra effort of explaining to the patient the long-term benefits of orthodontically repositioning teeth and, if necessary, should enthusiastically direct the patient to the specialist.[4]

THE RESTORATIVE OPTION

Restorative space management (RSM), is the alternative, or adjunctive, treatment modality to orthodontics in the management of the crowded dentition. The advent of advanced enamel and dentin adhesives and highly esthetic resin and ceramic materials, has made possible truly amazing esthetic results through tooth preparation and restoration.[4] In selected cases, RSM can be used to provide an esthetic outcome by strategic removal of tooth structure and the addition, either directly or indirectly, of composite and ceramic materials. The benefits of RSM include not only the apparent correction of tooth position but also real improvement in shape, size, discoloration removal, caries elimination, and replacement of defective restorations. The result is improved appearance and improved intraoral health.[3,13] Careful evaluations of periodontal health and gingival architecture, structural support for proposed restorations, occlusion, and esthetics, are the details to be considered in the decision tree of whether or not to opt for an RSM approach to the correction of the crowded dentition. The foregoing analysis leads to a determination as to whether RSM alone, orthodontics alone, or a combination of both is the best approach to achieve patient goals.[9,13]

PERIODONTAL CONSIDERATION

Irregular alignment of teeth, commonly found in cases of malocclusion, can make plaque control difficult.[14] Restoration contour is also extremely important to the maintenance of periodontal health.[14] Restorations that promote periodontal instability, encourage food impaction, retain plaque, and impede proper oral hygiene are contraindicated.[3,14] Esthetics requires that the relationship between gingival levels and tooth appearance, the balance of pink to white, must be considered.[4] In dental crowding, the more labially inclined teeth have a thinner gingiva, a shallower sulcus, and margins positioned more apically.[3,9] The opposite applies to lingually positioned teeth, for which thicker gingiva, deeper sulcus, and margins positioned more coronally are the rule.[3,9] Papillae levels are another important consideration. Interdental papillae conform to the interdental embrasure form. Because of the presence of excessively small interdental embrasures, the papillae in crowded dentitions are located apically.[9] The pleasing appearance of pink tissue that is healthy and symmetric is influenced by all of these factors. Negative gingival and interdental papillae architecture cannot be corrected through RSM alone.[3] Gingivectomy, osseous crown lengthening, and apically positioned flap surgery are periodontal therapies that can correct gingival margins in the crowded dentition.[3,9] In the treatment planning process, an acceptable position of the most apical gingival margin (typically on the buccally positioned tooth), indicates that surgical correction of the asymmetry on the lingually positioned teeth is needed.[3,9] Mild to moderate discrepancies are surgically easy to manage. Orthodontics is indicated in severe asymmetry if aggressive periodontal therapy may compromise tooth stability or retention.[8] Periodontal surgery cannot increase the height of interproximal bone or predictably grow interproximal tissue. Therefore, severe crowding, in which papillae disharmony is pronounced, requires the benefits obtained from orthodontic treatment.[9,15]

BIOLOGIC AND STRUCTURAL LIMITATIONS

The treatment of every case of crowding is a challenge, especially when the restorative option is chosen. In the crowded case, to align teeth with restorations such as veneers, more tooth reduction on selected teeth is needed than in the case presenting without crowding. There are limits to the degree of tooth structure that can be removed before pulpal and periodontal violation results.[3] Excessive tooth removal to accomplish the esthetic goals of therapy may require mutilation of the remaining tooth structure, thereby compromising the biologic and structural outcomes from 3 essential aspects: endodontic instability regarding questionable pulpal health and the long-term prognosis of root canal treatment; structural instability of the remaining tooth structure to support the restoration and occlusal scheme; and periodontal instability caused by changes in restorative tooth morphology.[3]

The structural integrity of a labially positioned tooth, which typically needs a significant amount of labial reduction to bring it into the desired position, may be severely compromised. Lingually positioned teeth require significant lingual reduction to compensate for excessively thick incisal edges.[9] The long-term survival of rotated teeth, which need reduction buccolingually on both the mesial and distal aspects,[9] influences the amount of tooth reduction.[5] The more conservative a tooth preparation, the better the structural support to the intended restoration.[3,9] In addition, overaggressive preparation leads to bonding on dentin as opposed to the more predictable enamel.[5]

OCCLUSAL FACTORS

Regardless of the esthetics achieved, whether through orthodontics, RSM, or a combination of the two, the postrestorative occlusion must be stable.[16] If a stable occlusion is perceived as esthetically unacceptable, careful attention should be given to avoid converting a stable occlusion into an unstable occlusion in the restorative esthetic correction. The common signs of a stable occlusion are healthy temperomandibular joint, firm teeth, no excessive wear, teeth that do not move from their position, and supporting structures that can be maintained in a healthy condition.[16] The crowded dentition can present with varying occlusal patterns such as increased or decreased overjet and overbite. These malocclusions can be a challenge because of spatial discrepancies and the ability to resolve them restoratively. RSM of anterior crowding is intimately associated with canine and incisal guidance. Therefore, an occlusal analysis should be included in the treatment planning process.[9,17] Although some patients with open bites, cross bites, and deep bites can present with an occlusion as stable as those with an ideal occlusion, these cases require careful analysis. If the crowded case can also benefit from the inclusion of anterior centric stops and enhanced anterior guidance, the best option, RSM (additive/reshaping) or orthodontics (repositioning), must be clearly identified.[9,16] Crowded teeth are often unstable because of a lack of centric holding contacts. Teeth without an antagonistic stop or a substitute, such as the tongue, tend to supererupt. If a planned restoration shortens an extruded tooth, and a centric stop does not provide it, it will tend to supererupt again.[7]

The envelope of function must also be considered when planning a change in tooth morphology intended to enhance esthetics. The neurologically programmed tooth closure pattern may be interfered with when altering the buccal surface of lower teeth or lingual surface of upper teeth.[11] The mandible has favored pathways of motion. If restored teeth interfere with these patterns, the result will be occlusal instability. Signs of instability may include fremitus, excessive wear on the labioincisal contours of lower teeth or the lingual contours of upper incisors, tooth movement, or fracture of anterior laminate restorations.[18] Proper occlusal diagnosis of the crowded dentition ensures that the alignment correction is routed properly during the treatment planning, and the options of restorative, orthodontics, or a combination of both is weighed so a more predictable esthetic and functional result is achieved.

ESTHETIC CONSIDERATIONS

Tooth shade, proportion, size, and positioning to conform to an adequate arch form are the esthetic goals included in the RSM of crowded cases.[3,7,13] For patients presenting with crowded teeth that will need to be restored after orthodontic treatment, regardless of the success of the orthodontic treatment, restorative correction alone should be considered. Inability to achieve the desired tooth shade by bleaching, or inadequate tooth size and shape, are indications for the correction of crowding by RSM alone.[9] RSM is a good option in mild to moderate cases,[3] in which the malposition discrepancy permits less tooth structure preparation, allows for better restoration contours, and the periodontal remodeling, if needed, is minimally invasive.[9] Patients managed with restorative correction do not risk unstable outcomes with orthodontic relapse, especially in the long-term retention of rotational corrections common in crowded dentitions treated orthodontically.[3,9]

The key tool in determining appropriate esthetic outcome is the diagnostic waxup or setup.[9] The size, shape, and position of the maxillary central incisors are the most influential factors in a harmonious anterior dentition.[3,19] Ward identified the recurring esthetic dental proportion, which is the width-to-length proportion of teeth, and is usually between 75% and 80%. To calculate the ideal width for any tooth use the formula $W = L \times 0.80$.[2,10] Caution should be observed in using mathematical tools to determine tooth proportions in crowded dentitions. For example, the golden proportion can be a useful tool for doing waxups. However, it can fail to create ideal esthetics in patients with diastemata or crowding. The golden proportion creates a proportion relative to the tooth width only. This limitation can create a problem. Creating an ideal proportion only for the central incisors may be more pleasing, allowing the lateral incisors minor differences. The laterals are less noticeable and look good provided they have symmetry.[9] There is no formula that can guarantee to obtain harmony and an ideal anterior dentition. In crowded cases, the patients own perception, the clinical limitations, and the available resources must be considered to achieve the best possible outcome.

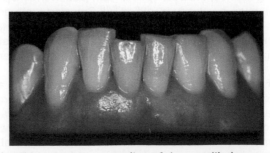

Fig. 4. Patient with mild to moderate crowding of the mandibular anteriors.

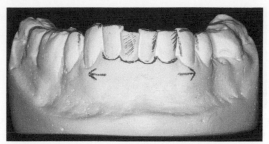

Fig. 5. Midfacial gingival heights are marked in red; areas of proposed tooth width reduction are marked in blue to allow subsequent expansion of the arch form.

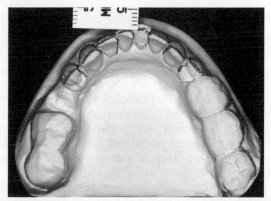

Fig. 6. Red lines mark the ideal arch form on the preoperative model. Approximately 1 mm of buccolingual overlap was evident and mesiodistal overlap of less than 1 mm.

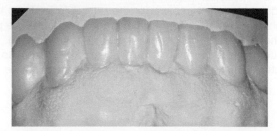

Fig. 7. A diagnostic waxup was created to visualize the postoperative tooth form and to fabricate preparation guides.

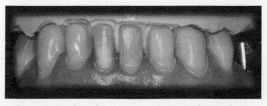

Fig. 8. Tooth preparations viewed with a preparation guide in place.

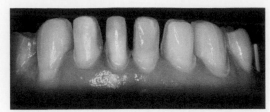

Fig. 9. Preparations for porcelain laminate veneers and full coverage on endodontically treated lower right incisor.

CLINICAL PROCEDURES FOR CROWDING

A 49-year-old woman presented with mild to moderate misalignment of teeth numbers 22 to 27. Tooth 25 was discolored and necrotic. Although tooth 24 was mesially rotated, tooth 25 was positioned facially, creating an uneven overlapping appearance (**Fig. 4**).

The mandibular arch was evaluated to ensure proper incisal contours. Following impression capture, a stone cast was fabricated. Areas that required reduction were marked in blue, and red lines were drawn on the incisal edges to indicate the ideal arch position. The free gingival tissue height was also marked in red to ensure development of the correct gingival architecture. This class I case showed little visible free gingival margin distortion.

The mesiodistal areas of reduction were marked in blue to allow proper arch expansion of the restored dental arch. Red marks on the facial aspect of teeth 23, 24, and 25 indicated areas of reduction to restoratively shift the labiality positioned teeth lingually (**Figs. 5** and **6**). A diagnostic wax-up was used as the basis for the preparation guides (**Fig. 7**). Using silicone putty, an incisal index of the waxup was made. Proper tooth reduction was required to create space for the porcelain laminate veneers, except for tooth 25, which was prepared for a full coverage zirconium core porcelain crown after root canal therapy and postcore preparation (**Figs. 8** and **9**). Once the tooth preparation was completed, an impression was made and sent to the laboratory. The definitive restorations were cemented using a resin adhesive and composite cement (**Fig. 10**).

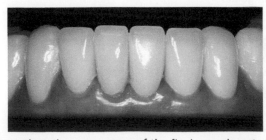

Fig. 10. Immediate postinsertion appearance of the final ceramic restorations.

SUMMARY

A careful analysis of patients with dental crowding is necessary to choose the role orthodontics is to play in corrective treatment. For most patients, at least some orthodontic therapy is appropriate. It is the responsibility of the treating dentist to understand the implications and the prognosis in any proposed treatment plan and communicate with the patient in a manner that ensures that the patient fully understands the implications of therapy. The long-term health of the patient must always be the first consideration. To promote cosmetics and ease of treatment to the same level as patient welfare would be a backward step for the profession. The argument that it is the patient who ultimately has the right to decide the course of treatment does not relieve the practitioner from the responsibility of doing no harm.

REFERENCES

1. Barnabe E, Del Castillho CE, Flores-Mir C. Intra-arch occlusal indicators of crowding in the permanent dentition. Am J Orthod Dentofacial Orthop 2005; 17(1):19–25.
2. Bernabe E, Villanueva KM, Flores-Mir C. Tooth width ratios in crowded and non-crowded dentitions. Angle Orthod 2004;74(6):756–8.
3. Gurel G, Chu S, Kim J. Restorative space management. In: Tarnow D, Chu S, Kim J, editors. Aesthetic restorative dentistry principles and practice. Mahwah (NJ): Quintessence; 2008. p. 405–25.
4. Heymann HO, Kokich VG. Orthodontics: viable treatment option or "Quick fix" cop-out. J Esthet Restor Dent 2002;14(5):263–4.
5. Jacobson N, Frank CA. The myth of instant orthodontics: an ethical quandary. J Am Dent Assoc 2008;139(4):424–34.
6. Spear FM, Kokich VG, Mathews DP. Interdisciplinary management of anterior esthetics. J Am Dent Assoc 2006;137(2):160–9.
7. Dawson P. Treating crowded, irregular or interlocking anterior teeth. In: Dawson P, editor. Functional occlusion from TMJ to smile design. Missouri: Mosby; 2007. p. 525–45.
8. Celenza F. Restorative—orthodontic interrelationships. In: Tarnow D, Chu S, Kim J, editors. Aesthetic restorative dentistry principles and practice. Mahwah (NJ): Mosby; 2008. p. 427–57.
9. Spear FM. The esthetic correction of anterior dental mal-alignment conventional vs. instant (restorative) orthodontics. J Calif Dent Assoc 2004;32(2):133–41.
10. Fillion D. Adult orthodontics: problems and solutions with lingual orthodontics. In: Romano R, editor. The art of the smile. Integrating prosthodontics, orthodontics, periodontics, dental technology and plastic surgery in esthetic dental treatment. UK: Quintessence; 2005. p. 211–29.
11. Gurel G. Adjunctive orthodontics as related to periodontics and aesthetic dentistry. In: Gurel G, editor. The science and art of PLV. New Malden (UK): Quintessence; 2003. p. 417–44.
12. Alexander RG. Considerations in creating a beautiful smile. In: Romano R, editor. The art of the smile. Integrating prosthodontics, orthodontics, periodontics, dental technology and plastic surgery in esthetic dental treatment. UK: Quintessence; 2005. p. 187–210.
13. Kim J, Chu S, Gürel G, et al. Restorative space management: treatment planning and clinical considerations for insufficient space. Pract Proced Aesthet Dent 2005;17(1):19–25.

14. Hinrichs JE. The role of dental calculus and other predisposing factors. In: Carranza NT, editor. Clinical periodontology. Danvers (MA): Saunders; 2002. p. 182–203.
15. Kokich VG. The role of orthodontics as an adjunct to periodontal therapy. In: Carranza NT, editor. Clinical periodontology. Danvers (MA): Saunders; 2002. p. 704–18.
16. Dawson P. Requirements for occlusal stability. In: Dawson P, editor. Functional occlusion from TMJ to smile design. Missouri: Mosby; 2007. p. 345–8.
17. Dawson P. Solving occlusal problems through programmed treatment planning. In: Dawson P, editor. Functional occlusion from TMJ to smile design. Missouri: Mosby; 2007. p. 349–63.
18. Gurel G. Porcelain - bonded restoration and function. In: Gurel G, editor. The science and art of PLV. New Malden (UK): Quintessence; 2003. p. 135–55.
19. Gurel G. Smile design. In: Gurel G, editor. The science and art of PLV. New Malden (UK): Quintessence; 2003. p. 59–112.

Cements and Adhesives for All-Ceramic Restorations

Adriana P. Manso, DDS, MSc, PhD[a,b],
Nelson R.F.A. Silva, DDS, MSc, PhD[c],
Estevam A. Bonfante, DDS, MSc, PhD[d], Thiago A. Pegoraro, DDS, PhD[e],
Renata A. Dias, DDS[c], Ricardo M. Carvalho, DDS, PhD[f,*]

KEYWORDS

- Dental cements • Esthetic dentistry • Resin-based cements
- Simplified adhesives systems • Incompatibility • Ceramics
- Silanation

Dental luting cements are designed to retain restorations, appliances, and post and cores in a stable and, presumably, long-lasting position in the oral environment. Retention mechanisms are reported to be chemical, mechanical (friction), and micro-mechanical (hybridized tissue), but they are usually a combination of two or three mechanisms, depending on the nature of the cement and of the substrate. Among dental luting cements commercially available, there are resin-based and nonresin-based cements. They must have for their acceptable clinical performance adequate resistance to dissolution, strong bond through mechanical interlocking and adhesion, high strength under tension, good manipulation properties, and also be biologically compatible with the substrate.[1,2]

Traditionally, zinc phosphate cement has been regarded as the most popular material, despite its disadvantages as low hardness, solubility and lack of adhesion.[3]

This work was partially supported by Cap grants # 300305/0-4, Brazil, and FAPESP # 04/1263-0, and # 2010/06152-9 Brazil.

[a] Department of Operative Dentistry, University of Florida, College of Dentistry, 1600 Archer Road, Gainesville, FL 32610, USA

[b] Instituto HNary, Al. Octávio Pinheiro Brisola, 12-67, 17012-901, Bauru, São Paulo, Brazil

[c] Department of Prosthodontics, New York University College of Dentistry, 345 East 24th Street, New York, NY 10010, USA

[d] Department of Prosthodontics, UNIGRANRIO University, School of Dentistry, Rio de Janeiro, Brazil

[e] Department of Prosthodontics, University Center, CESMAC, Rua Cônego Machado, 918, Farol, Maceio, Alagoas, 57051160, Brazil

[f] Department of Prosthodontics, University of São Paulo, Bauru School of Dentistry, Al. Otávio P. Brisola 9-75, Bauru, São Paulo 17012901, Brazil

* Corresponding author. Departamento de Prótese, Al. Otávio P. Brisola 9-75, Bauru, São Paulo 17012901, Brazil.

E-mail address: ricfob@fob.usp.br

doi:10.1016/j.cden.2011.01.011
0011-8532/11/$ – see front matter © 2011 Elsevier Inc. All rights reserved.

Although the final marginal accuracy of all-ceramic systems processes (computer-aided design [CAD]/computer-aided manufacturing [CAM] especially) have significantly improved, these still result in larger internal gaps than cast crowns, possibly resulting in thicker cement layers[4] and poorer frictional retention to the abutments. These would be critical challenges for zinc phosphate cement because of its solubility and lack of adhesiveness. Although zinc–phosphate has been indicated for some all-ceramic systems (ca In-Ceram [VITA Zahnfabrik H. Rauter GmbH & Co KG, Bad Säckingen, Germany], Procera [Nobel Biocare, Switzerland], Cercon [DeguDent, Hanau, Germany], Lava [3M ESPE, St Paul, MN, USA]), long-term clinical data are yet to be published.

Glass ionomer cements are also of great interest for clinicians. These cements exhibit several clinical advantages,[5] including physicochemical bonding to tooth structures,[5,6] long-term fluoride release, and low coefficients of thermal expansion.[5,7] However, their low mechanical strength compromises their use in high-stress-bearing areas.[5,8] Glass ionomer cements can be used to cement core-reinforced ceramics such as those also allowed to be cemented with zinc phosphate. However, glass ionomer cements would not suit well for ceramics requiring support from the cement. Therefore resin-based cements have become popular, because they have the potential to address the disadvantages of solubility, support, and lack of adhesion described for previous materials.[1]

Restorative dentistry constantly undergoes changes, and no currently available cement is ideal for all situations. The advent of adhesive luting cements has considerably expanded the scope of fixed prosthodontics. This article will focus on resin-based cements as luting agent for all-ceramic systems, due to the important role the cement plays in the final clinical success of such treatment modality.

RESIN CEMENTS AND ADHESIVE INTERFACES

Resin cements have become popular clinically because of their ability to bond both the tooth structure and restoration. Bonded indirect restorations constitute a substantial part of contemporary dentistry.[9] The successful use of resin cements depends on several aspects related to the bonding mechanisms to both dental tissues and restorations. The scientific knowledge of the materials currently available as well as the acknowledgment of their limitations and indications are key factors for durable restorations. Several new luting cements and ceramic systems have been introduced in the last few years, and their chemistry and structural characteristics are fundamental to produce an optimal and reliable bonding to both tooth and restoration interfaces.

Resin Cements: Chemistry and Properties

Table 1 summarizes various resin-based cements with their respective characteristics and chemical compositions.

Resin-based luting cements were primarily based on acrylic resin chemistry. Their subsequent development, however, has been based on the chemistry of resin composites and adhesives.[10] Currently, several new resin cements are available in the market. These are offered in a wide variety of bonding mechanisms, curing modes, indications, and features (see **Table 1**). The choice of a particular resin cement requires understanding of the material's characteristics as well as how it performs individually and integrated in the restorative system. There are two main categories of resin luting cements: the conventional resin luting cements, which have no inherent adhesion to tooth structure and require a bonding agent, and the self-adhesive resin cements, which do not require a separate bonding treatment to the dental substrate.

Conventional resin luting cements

Since the 1970s, resin cements have been formulated based on dimethacrylate resin chemistry as two-paste systems, which are easy to mix and cure at room temperature.[3] Their bonding to tooth structure relies on the use of etch-and-rinse or self-etch adhesives. Composition is usually a mixture of dimethacrylate monomers, inorganic fillers (60% to 70% by weight), and initiator. Silica or high molecular weight oligomers may also be added to modify the rheological properties and achieve optimum handling characteristics. Examples of their clinical applications include metal-based crowns and bridges, zirconia and alumina framed crowns, fiber posts, and cast metal post and core. Because of the importance of light- and dual-curing systems, a separate topic was created to address their clinical application and polymerization mechanisms.

Curing protocols and its clinical relevance

Light-cured Conventional resin cements can be exclusively light-cured. When comparing cements, light-cure products offer the clinical advantages of extended working time, setting on demand, and improved color stability. However, the use of light-cure only cements is limited to situations such as cementing veneers or shallow inlays, where the thickness and color of the restoration do not affect the ability of the curing light to polymerize the cement.[11,12]

Dual-cured Dual-cured resin cements are often provided in two-paste systems (see **Table 1**). Dual-cure resin cements are indicated when delivering restorations where material characteristics may inhibit sufficient light energy from being transmitted to the cement.[13] In these situations, light intensity reaching the cement may be sufficient to trigger the light-activated polymerization process, but a self-polymerized catalyst is needed to ensure maximal cure. The delivery method usually involves mixing of paste to paste (see **Table 1**). One of the pastes contains a reducing amine and a photo initiator. The other paste contains peroxide, usually benzoyl peroxide. In an interesting variation of the initiator system, the anaerobic cements begin polymerization only when the ambient oxygen supply is cut off after placement of the prosthetic device. This feature provides extended working and setting times and offers easy removal of excess materials.[14,15] Although the dual-curing concept seems to be attractive, several issues have been brought up in the dental literature regarding its performance, and these concerns are going to be addressed throughout the text.

Little has been published on the light-curing potential of dual-cure cements. While earlier research suggests that auto-cure alone is not sufficient to achieve maximum cement hardening,[16,17] recent literature indicates that the curing kinetics of dual-cure resin cements is more complex than previously thought.[18] Studies indicate that light-activating some dual-cure cements appears to interfere with the self-cure mechanism and restrict the cement from achieving its maximum mechanical properties.[19,20]

Some dual-cure cements show their self-curing mechanism to be somehow limited when immediately light-activated in the dual-cure mode. This limitation may compromise the final mechanical properties of the resin cements.[19] This information is of great importance for the clinical practice, since light activation is always recommended by the manufacturer. It remains to be demonstrated whether the same phenomenon occurs with all resin-based cement systems. While such information is not available, it is advisable to delay the light-curing procedure of dual-cure cements to the maximum time clinically possible.[20] In this way, self-curing progress will be further along, to a point when light activation no longer interferes with the self-curing kinetics. The ideal time frame between mixing and the light-activation has not yet been determined, but some studies have shown that light-curing 5 to 10 minutes after mixing

Table 1
Representative resin cement systems

Products	Company	Adhesive	Delivery	Curing	Composition
Bistite II DC	Tokuyama (Tokyo, Japan)	Primer 1A+ 1B/primer 2	Paste/paste	Dual	Silica-zirconia (77% weight) filler, dimethacrylate, MAC-10 (adhesive promoter), initiator
Calibra	Dentsply/Caulk (Milford, DE, USA)	Prime and bond NT	Paste/paste	Dual	Base: barium boron fluoralumino silicate glass, bis-phenol A diglycidyldimethacrylate, polymerizable dimethacrylate resin, hydrophobic amorphopus silica, titanium dioxide, di-camphoroquinon. Catalyst: barium boron fluoralumino silicate glass, bis-phenol A diglycidyldimethacrylate, polymerizable dimethacrylate resin, hydrophobic amorphopus silica, titanium dioxide, benzoyl peroxide
C&B Cement	Bisco (Schaumburg, IL, USA)	All-bond 2 one step	Paste/paste dual syringe	Self	Base: Bis-GMA, ethoxylated bis-gma, triethelenegycol dimethacrylate, fused silica, glass filler, sodium fluoride. Catalyst: Bis-GMA, triethelenegycol dimethacrylate, fused silica
Choice 2	Bisco	All-bond/one step	Paste	Light	Strontium glass, amorphous silica, Bis-GMA
Duo-Link	Bisco	All-bond 2 one step/plus	Paste/paste dual syringe; automix	Dual	Base: Bis-GMA, triethyleneglycol dimethacrylate, urethane dimethacrylate, glass filler Catalyst: Bis-GMA, triethyleneglycol dimethacrylate, glass filler
BisCem	Bisco	Self-adhesive	Paste/paste dual syringe; automix	Dual	Bis (hydroxyethyl methacrylate) phosphate (base), tetraethylene glycol dimethacrylate, dental glass

Product	Manufacturer	System	Delivery/mix	Polymerization	Composition
NX 3 Nexus	Kerr (Washington, DC, USA)	Optibond solo plus optibond all-in-one	Paste/paste dual syringe; automix	Dual	Uncured methacrylate ester monomers, nonhazardous inert mineral fillers, nonhazardous activators and stabilizers, and radiopaque agent
Maxcem	Kerr	Self-adhesive	Paste/paste dual syringe; automix	Dual	GPDM (glycerol dimethacrylate dihydrogen phosphate), comonomers (mono-, di-, and tri-functional methacrylate monomers), stabilizer, barium glass fillers, fluoroaluminosilicate glass filler, fumed silica (filler load 67% weight, particle size 3.6 μm
Super Bond C&B	Sun Medical (Grand Prairie, TX, USA)	Monomer/catalyst V/polymer powder	4 drops of monomer/1 drop of catalyst s/1 small cup of standard measuring spoon	Self	MMA (methyl methacrylate), 4-methacryloxyethyl trimellitate anhydride (4-META), tri-nbutylborane (TBB- catalyst)
Clearfil Esthetic Cement	Kuraray (Tokyo, Japan)	Self-etch DC bond system	Paste/paste dual syringe; automix	Dual	Paste A: bis-phenol A diglycidylmethacrylate, TEGMA, methacrylate monomers, silanated glass filler, colloidal silica; Paste B: bis-phenol A diglycidylmethacrylate, TEGMA, methacrylate monomers, silanated glass filler, silanated silica, colloidal silica, benzoyl peroxide, CQ, pigments

(continued on next page)

Table 1
(continued)

Products	Company	Adhesive	Delivery	Curing	Composition
Panavia F 2.0	Kuraray	ED primer	Paste/paste	Dual	Paste A: 10-methacryloyloxydecyl, dihydrogen phosphate, hydrophobic aromatic dimethacrylate, hydrophobic aliphatic dimethacrylate, hydrophilic aliphatic dimethacrylate, silanated silica filler, silanated colloidal silica, dl-camphorquinone, catalysts, initiators Paste B: hydrophobic aromatic dimethacrylate, hydrophobic aliphatic, dimethacrylate, hydrophilic aliphatic dimethacrylate, silanated barium glass filler, catalysts, accelerators, pigments
Breeze	Pentron Clinical Tech (Orange, CA, USA)	Self-adhesive	Paste/paste dual syringe; automix	Dual	Mixture of bis-GMA, UDMA, TEG-DMA, HEMA, and 4-MET resins, silane-treated bariumborosilicate glasses, silica initiators, stabilizers and UV absorber, organic and/or inorganic pigments, opacifiers
GCem	GC (Tokyo, Japan)	Self-adhesive	Capsules	Dual	Powder: fluoroaminosilicate glass, initiator, pigment Liquid: 4-MET, phosphoric acid ester monomer, water, UDMA, dimethacrylate, silica powder, initiator, stabilizer
Embrace WetBond	Pulpdent (Watertown, MA, USA)	Self-adhesive	Standard syringe or automix	Dual	Uncured acrylate resins, amorphous silica, sodium fluoride
MonoCem	Shofu Dental (San Marcos, CA, USA)	Self-adhesive	Paste/paste dual syringe; automix	Dual	Not available

Multilink Sprint	Ivoclar/Vivadent (Schaan, Principality of Liechtenstein)	Paste/paste dual syringe; automix	Self-adhesive	Dual	Dimethacrylates and acidic monomers, barium glass, ytterbium trifluoride, silicon dioxide, mean particle size is 5 μm, total volume of inorganic fillers is ~48%
Multilink	Ivoclar/Vivadent	Paste/paste dual syringe; automix	Primer A + B	Self	Dimethacrylate and HEMA, barium glass filler, silicon dioxide filler, ytterbium trifluoride, catalysts and stabilizers, pigments
Variolink II	Ivoclar/Vivadent	Paste/paste	Excite adhesive	Dual	Paste of dimethacrylates, inorganic fillers, ytterbiumtrifluoride, initiators, stabilizers and pigments; (Bis-GMA, triethylene glycoldimethacrylate, urethanedimethacrylate, benzoyl peroxide)
Rely X ARC	3M ESPE (St Paul, MN, USA)	Paste/paste; clicker	Adper single bond	Dual	Bisphenol-A-diglycidylether dimethacrylate (BisGMA), triethylene glycol dimethacrylate (TEGDMA), polymer, zirconia/silica filler, filler loading approximately 67.5% by weight, particle size for the filler is 1.5μm.
Rely X Unicem	3M ESPE	Capsules (Aplicap: 0.01 mL; Maxicap: 0.36 mL)	Self-adhesive	Dual	Powder: glass fillers, silica, calcium hydroxide, self-curing initiators, pigments, light-curing initiators (filler load 72% weight, particle size <9.5 μm); Liquid: methacrylated phosphoric esters, dimethacrylates, acetate, stabilizers, self-curing initiators
Rely X Unicem	3M ESPE	Paste/paste; Clicker	Self-adhesive	Dual	Glass powder, methacrylated phosphoric acid esters, triethylene glycol dimethacrylate (TEG-DMA), silane treated silica, sodium persulfate

does not seem to interfere with final cure and properties, at least for most of the cements evaluated.[19]

It is interesting to note that there is no direct correlation between alterations in the degree of conversion (DC) caused by different curing modes and changes in the mechanical properties of the resin cements.[19] The lack of linear correlation between DC, properties, and density of crosslink in the polymer has also been reported elsewhere.[21] However, cements that do not cure properly with light activation or have a compromised self-cure reaction may experience adverse chemical reactions and permeability issues when associated with simplified adhesive systems.[20] This clinically implies that the longer the resin cement takes to set, the greater will be the chance of adverse effects when coupling resin cements to simplified adhesives. To overcome these problems, clinicians have been advised to use three-step etch and rinse or two-step self-etch adhesives.[20,22–24] When using these systems, adverse chemical reaction and permeability are prevented by the nonacidic and relatively higher hydrophobic characteristics of the bonding resin that comprise the last step of the application of such systems.[22] Clinical trials are necessary to demonstrate how these issues may affect the long-term performance of different combinations of adhesives and cements.

Concerns on mixing and working time of dual-cure cements Resin-based cements are formulated to provide the handling characteristics required for particular applications. The setting mechanism of dual-cure resin cements is usually based on redox reaction of benzoyl peroxide with aromatic tertiary amines (represented by catalyst and base paste, respectively). At least one paste contains the light-sensitive compound (camphorquinone [CQ]) responsible for initiating the light-cure setting mechanism. After the pastes are mixed together, and until light is provided, the working time is controlled by the ratio between inhibitors of the self-curing reaction and the amount of peroxide and aromatic tertiary amines. Both inhibitors and peroxides are organic chemical compounds susceptible to degradation upon storage. Therefore, dual-cure resin cements have a limited shelf-life and the setting mechanism of those cements may fluctuate during that time, depending on the conditions of storage that might alter the reactive potential of such components. In vitro evidences indicate that both working time (WT) and setting time (ST) may be significantly altered upon storage,[19] particularly if the storage temperature is far above the recommended (> 18°–22°C). In one study, some cements presented shortened WT/ST, while others presented extended WT/ST after the kits were purposely aged for 12 weeks at 37°C.[19] This occurred because of the instability of the components during storage. Degradation of peroxide would extend the WT/ST, and degradation of inhibitors would shorten them. The implications of such changes on the mechanical properties of the resin cements are yet unclear. However, clinicians handling resin cements with shortened WT may experience some clinical difficulties when luting multiple crowns, for example. Conversely, increased adverse chemical reaction and permeability problems may be expected for resin cements with extended WT and ST used in combination with an acidic and permeable simplified adhesive system. This is mostly because the extended ST allows the uncured cement longer time in contact with the acidic adhesive, thus prolonging the adverse reaction.

Bonding mechanisms and incompatibility issues of dual-cure cements Most adhesive systems used with resin-based cements are simplified adhesive systems, because of clinical trends for reduced steps during adhesive procedures. These simplified adhesives are basically of two types: the etch-and-rinse, single-bottle systems and the all-in-one self-etch adhesives. They are both somewhat acidic and hydrophilic in nature.

During cementation, the acidic groups in the uncured layer of simplified adhesive agents (due to presence of oxygen) compete with peroxides for aromatic tertiary amines of the luting agent, resulting in an acid–base reaction between the adhesive and the resin cement. This reaction minimizes proper copolymerization between the two, and the longer the cement takes to cure, the more extent is the compromising effect.[25–27] Additionally, the hydrophilic characteristics of such adhesive systems function as permeable membranes. This hydrophilic behavior permits the flux of water through the adhesive after polymerization.[28,29] The presence of water at the interface between the adhesive and the cement compromises the total bonded area and proper polymerization of the cement. Water droplets may accumulate at the interface and then function as stress raisers, leading to failure of the adhesive–cement interface (**Fig. 1**).[28] This permeability problem could be partially solved by the application of an intermediate layer of a relatively more hydrophobic, nonacidic low viscosity resin separating the acidic layer of adhesive from the composite resin cement.[28,30] The water that accumulates at the interface derives from the hydrated dentin underneath. The negative effect of such water permeation on the bond strength of resin cements to dentin could be confirmed in in vitro studies.[28,29] Those studies demonstrated improved bond strengths when the teeth were purposely dehydrated in ascending ethanol series before bonded. As such dehydration of dentin is impossible to achieve in daily practice, clinicians are advised to use less permeable adhesive systems such as three-step etch and rinse or two-step self-etch when bonding self- or dual-cured resin cements to dentin.[28,30] The major advantage of these systems is that they include a layer of a relatively more hydrophobic and nonacidic resin as the third or second step. This additional layer will not cause adverse reaction with the basic amines of the cement and will reduce the permeability of the adhesive layer.[31,32] The incompatibility issue has brought up concerns for several clinical procedures. The worst clinical scenario would occur when luting posts using simplified adhesives associated with dual-cured resin cements (see **Fig. 1**). Proper bonding to the apical portion might be severely compromised by the adverse interactions between adhesive and luting composite due to a lack of light exposure. Without light activation, dual-cure resin cements will actually function as exclusively self-cure cements. In this mode, the cement will take longer to cure, and this allows more time for the adverse reaction and transudation of water from dentin to occur. A similar situation occurs when the cement takes longer to set because of alterations in the WT/ST caused by inadequate storage conditions, as described previously. Based on those limitations, some studies have suggested the development of a specific bonding system for this purpose.[31,32] Recent studies have shown that the push-out resistance of posts luted with resin cements was similar, regardless of the use of adhesive systems to bond to root dentin.[31,32] A more predictable, truly adhesive luting procedure can only be achieved when clinicians combine the use of resin cements with three-step etch and rinse or two-step self-etch bonding systems. Self-adhesive resin cements have been strongly recommended to lute posts and crowns as an alternative to conventional luting systems, avoiding incompatibility and permeability issues due to wrong combinations of adhesives and cements.

When cementing inlays, onlays, and crowns, immediate dentin sealing concept[33] may be a useful clinical alternative to overcome the incompatibility and permeability issues. Further details on this approach can be found elsewhere.[20,34,35]

Self-adhesive resin cements

The simplification to only one step of resin luting procedures was achieved with the self-adhesive resin cements.[36] This system uses a dual-cure concept for polymerization, and no pretreatments using bonding agents on the tooth surface is required,

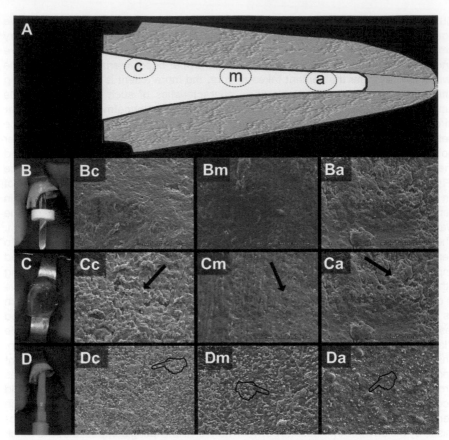

Fig. 1. This sequence of micrographs shows the in vivo morphologic characteristics of root dentin during postcementation procedures using an etch-and-rinse two-step adhesive system. Observations were made in (*A*) cervical, middle, and apical thirds (*dotted circles*) of the root canal by means of an impression with a polyvinyl siloxane material taken immediately after (*B*) postspace preparation, (*C*) etching with phosphoric acid, and (*D*) application of the adhesive system. The impression of the root canal was then positioned in a container allowing an epoxy resin to be poured covering up to half of the impression. After gold sputtering, the samples were taken to a scanning electron microscope at 1000 × magnification for evaluation. After postspace preparation, the anticipated presence of a smear layer (*arrows*) was observed in the (Bc) cervical and (Bm) middle thirds, but noticeably higher amounts were detected at the apical section (Ba). Remarkably, etching with phosphoric acid did not effectively remove the smear layer at either cervical, middle, or apical thirds (Cc, Cm, Ca, respectively), and dentinal tubules do not seem to be available for hybridization. Micrographs taken after subsequent layering of an adhesive system with a microbrush revealed evidence of water permeation and blistering (pointers) protruding from the dentin surface, and they were more frequently observed in (Dc) cervical and (Dm) middle thirds relative to the (Da) apical third. One possible reason may be the progressively lower number and diameter of dentinal tubules toward the apical area and the reduced permeability in this area.

making its application clinically attractive. Self-adhesive resin cements are claimed to be moisture-tolerant, to release fluoride, and to present no postoperative sensitivity.[37] Thus, all these factors combined fit to the clinical demand for simplification and less technique sensitiveness.[38]

The first of this class of materials was introduced as a powder–liquid material provided in unit–dose capsule that had to be triturated (RelyX Unicem [3M ESPE, St Paul, MN, USA]), and newer paste-paste versions have been commercialized (see **Table 1**). The setting reaction is initiated by light exposure and by the self-curing mechanism. In general, the initial low pH is neutralized through reactions between acid groups and alkaline filler and tooth apatite. Lower bond strengths to enamel compared with dentin have been reported, and this fact may limit the use of self-adhesive resin cements for bonding veneers.[15,38] Moreover, esthetic veneers and minimally invasive restorations require longer working time for positioning and demand more esthetic and shade availability than the ones that have been provided for self-adhesive kits.

Bonding mechanism of self-adhesive cements Conventional resin cements require an adhesive agent to mediate bonding to tooth structure, which can be either etch-and-rinse (three- or two-step) or self-etch adhesive system (two- or one-step). It seems that the more steps involved in the bonding procedure for both bonding approaches, the more stable is the bonded interface produced.[39] Conversely, when more clinical steps are required, it is also more critical to keep the bonding substrates properly isolated; additionally the chances are higher for technique sensitivity.

Self-adhesive resin cements do not require the bonding step. The acidity of the cement is strong enough to promote hybridization with the tooth structure. While still fluid, the acidic groups of the monomer dissolve the smear layer, which allows penetration of the cement into the dentinal tubules, thus providing a good hybrid layer and good adhesion. Micromechanical retention and chemical interaction between acidic groups and hydroxy-apatite are expected. It has been reported that self-adhesive cement showed chemical interaction with Ca ions derived from hydroxy-apatite.[40] Enamel bonding with a self-adhesive cement produced lower bond strengths than conventional resin cements but higher than glass–ionomer. It may be considered as an alternative to glass–ionomer luting cement for cementation of high-strength ceramic or metal-based restorations, but it might not be ideal for luting restorations such as veneers, inlays, and partial crowns if a considerable enamel surface area is present.[41] The use of phosphoric acid for etching enamel before the application of self-adhesive resin cement can result in bond strengths comparable to conventional resin cements.[42] However, previous etching can be detrimental for bond strengths to dentin.[43] Although self-adhesive and conventional resin cement–dentin interfaces are morphologically different,[43,44] self-adhesive cements have been reported to perform equally effective when compared with most conventional resin cements.[38,45,46] There is still a need for a more long-term clinical evaluation of self-adhesive cements.

Resin Cement and Water Sorption Phenomenon

When an all-ceramic crown is cemented, the assembly ceramic/cement/adhesive/tooth will be subjected to a watery environment. Resin cements should not only have low solubility, but also low water sorption because of esthetic and functional reasons.[47] The water sorption phenomenon has been demonstrated to have an important effect on the properties of resin cements after long periods of time.[48,49] Water sorption diminishes significantly the flexural strength of resin composites. The reduction of flexural strength as well as modulus of elasticity[50] may be critical for thick areas of resin cement. Scientific evidences show that absorbed water works as a plasticizer for the cements and, therefore, may create unsupported areas underneath restoration and consequently increase the chance of fracture of the restoration under mastication forces. Clinicians should keep as thin as possible the cement film to minimize the consequences of the plasticizing phenomenon for resin cements.[51] The water sorption may also result in hygroscopic expansion[50,52] of the cement, but the consequences of hygroscopic expansion on the long-term durability of dental cements, and consequently all-ceramic restoration, remain unknown.

Clinicians should be aware that cements that present extended working time or setting time, do not cure properly with light activation, or have a compromised self-cure mechanism will more severely suffer with hygroscopic expansion issues. Incomplete polymerization and nonconversion of monomer may result in loss of resin, and this may affect the biologic compatibility of the resin material.[53] Scientific evidence[54] has demonstrated that reducing the exposure time for polymerization of light-cure cements to 75% of that recommend by the manufacturer may facilitate fluid uptake and dissolution of the resin. Therefore, all measures should be taken to permit maximum polymerization of resin cements to minimize the water sorption phenomenon and its consequences.

Vrochari and collaborators[55] have recently evaluated water sorption and solubility of several cements. The authors observed that materials with similar polymerization mechanisms may perform differently during their interaction with water. Thus, clinicians are advised to be aware whether the resin-based cements to be chosen follow the International Organization for Standardization (ISO) standards regarding water sorption performance. Ideally, resin cements should present the lowest water sorption and solubility values possible.

Film Thickness of Resin-Based Cements

The importance of resin cement film thickness currently relies on the fact that most of the ceramic materials have considerable internal space. The effect of resin cement thickness on the fracture resistance of all-ceramic restorations is not completely established yet, but some studies have found some correlation between these factors. In 1994, Scherrer and colleagues[56] reported that when resin cement thickness of 300 μm or more was present, a gradual decrease of the fracture strength was observed[57] demonstrating that thick ceramic combined with minimal thickness of luting composite provided restorations with a favorable configuration with regard to prevent cracking.[57] It was also demonstrated that glass–ceramics with thick cement layers exhibit significantly lower reliability after water aging.[58] It seems that a thin cement thickness and proper bond to the ceramic structure is necessary for improved support and increased fracture resistance of all-ceramic crowns. Thicker cement layers have also been related to decreased bond strength of ceramic systems.[59] Thus, clinicians are strongly advised to maintain a minimal film thickness (approximately 50 μm) to minimize the effects of water sorption and its consequences to the properties of the cement and respective support for the ceramic restoration.

BONDING INTERFACE OF ALL-CERAMIC MATERIALS

The development of new cement and adhesive techniques expanded the use of ceramics and indirect resin composites in dentistry. Bonding ceramic materials to enamel and dentin combined with the improved strength of these indirect restorative materials has produced restorations with improved mechanical integrity and reduced risk for fracture.[60] Although a separate article of all-ceramic systems is included in this special issue for *Dental Clinics of North America*, a brief description of the ceramic materials characteristics will be presented to favor the understanding of their bonding strategies and mechanisms at the resin–cement/restorative material interface.

Glass Ceramics

Feldspathic glasses and Leucite-containing feldspathic glasses are still extensively used in veneers, inlays, and single anterior crowns. They offer excellent esthetic outcomes derived from their high translucency, fluorescence, and opalescence. However, these ceramics have drawbacks such as reduced strength and toughness. The glass–ceramic systems currently available are:

Leucite-reinforced glass-ceramics (sintered, hot-pressed or CAD-CAM) with flexural strengths of up to 120 MPa, which is considered to be sufficient for veneers, anterior crowns and posterior inlays

Fluormica glass-ceramics (CAD-CAM) with flexural strength of 120 to 150 MPa, which, combined with the adhesion to tooth tissues, may be adequate for selected posterior crowns.

A significant improvement of the mechanical properties (flexural strength around 350–450 MPa) of glass–ceramic systems was achieved with the development of lithium disilicate glass–ceramics (hot-pressed or CAD-CAM). Since the introduction of lithium disilicate ceramic to the market, the use of Leucite-reinforced glass–ceramics has declined. Moreover, besides the better mechanical properties and improved esthetic outcomes, high bond strength can be achieved when bonded to the tooth structure.[60]

High-Strength Polycrystalline Ceramics

Although high-strength polycrystalline ceramics (alumina and zirconia) broaden the applications of all-ceramic systems to posterior crowns and bridges, randomized clinical trials and clinical experience have been controversial regarding long-term survival.[61–67] As a result of its superior mechanical properties compared with alumina, zirconium became the first choice as a core or framework for all-ceramic restorations. However, it is imperative to mention that the bonding mechanisms to high-strength ceramics have been problematic as a result of lack of glass particles in its composition. This issue and possible adhesion options to high-strength ceramics are discussed in detail throughout the following section.

Bonding strategies for all-ceramic systems

The ability of a combination of resin cement/adhesive system to adhere to dental ceramics depends on the microstructure of the esthetic restoration and the surface treatment applied.[68] While roughening the surface by grinding or airborne particle abrasion is considered a way for improved adhesion for most of the esthetic materials, silanation appears to be only effective for silica-based ceramics.[69] A durable and reliable bond for dental resin-bonded ceramics is usually attempted via two principal mechanisms: (1) micromechanical attachment to porosities originated from hydrofluoric acid (HF) etching or (2) grit blasting, associated with a silane-coupling agent. Evaluations of bond strength between ceramic and resin composite have derived different conclusions about the effect of surface treatments. Controversy in the literature[70,71] relies on possible inefficacy or inactivity of the silane-coupling agent applied and operator's handling of the procedure. Meng and colleagues[72] recently demonstrated that hydrofluoric acid treatment could enhance the bond durability of resin/silanated glass ceramics, which might result from the increase of the chemical adhesion area on the ceramic rough surface and subsequently reduced degradation speed of the silane coupler, rather than the mechanical retention of the ceramic rough surface.[72]

Silane coupling

Silane-coupling agents are bi-functional molecules capable of bonding to the hydroxyl groups on ceramic surfaces and copolymerizing with the organic portion of the resin cement or adhesive. Silane primers contain a silane agent (usually γ-methacryloxypropyl-trimethoxy silane), a weak acid, and high amounts of solvents. To be effective, the silane agent must be hydrolyzed by the weak acid. Once hydrolyzed, silane primers have a limited shelf-life, and effectiveness progressively decays over time. The effectiveness of prehydrolyzed, single-bottle silane primers is, therefore, unpredictable if the user is not aware of when the solution was activated. Clinically, the only indicator seems to be the appearance of the liquid (ie, a clear solution is useful, while a milky-like solution should be discarded).[69] However, alcoholic solution (one-bottle systems) stays transparent, and the signs of alterations cannot be identified. Therefore, two-bottle solutions are preferred. Practitioners should strictly respect expiration date and follow the manufacturers' recommendations of silane systems.

The understanding of how the silanation process occurs on ceramic surfaces is of great importance to improve effectiveness of silanes. When a silane is applied to a ceramic surface and dried, three different structures are formed at what is called interphase layer.[73] The outermost layer consists of small oligomers that can be washed away by organic solvents or water at room temperature.[71] Closer to the glass surface, there is another layer of oligomers that is hydrolysable. To avoid hydrolysis of this layer after cementation, which could compromise the coupling of the cement with the ceramic, some authors recommend it be removed with hot water before bonding to silanated ceramic.[71,74] Attached to the glass there is a third layer, which is a monolayer that is covalently bonded to the silica phase of the ceramic and is hydrolytically stable.[70] This remaining monolayer of silane is not removed by these procedures, and it is responsible for the actual bond between the ceramic and the adhesive/cement system.

Since it is not possible to clinically control the application of a monolayer of silane, undesirable excess must be removed before bonding. This can be achieved by several methods. One way is to apply the silane followed by hot air drying (50°C $\pm$ 5°C) for 15 seconds for proper solvent evaporation. Then, rinse with hot water (80°C) for 15 seconds followed by another hot air drying for 15 seconds.[74] This procedure would eliminate water and solvent and wash away any unreacted silane (excess) primer components.[74] Alternatively, excess silane can be removed during the try-in step.

The try-in procedure is known to be a contaminant step. Therefore, it has been recommended to be done before silanation. Clinicians generally use the try-in step after receiving the surface-etched (hydrofluoric acid, HF) ceramic restoration from dental laboratories. However, the HF-treated ceramic surface is hydrophilic and more prone to be contaminated if the hydrophilic try-in paste is applied before the silanation step. Therefore, ceramic surfaces should be silanated before the try-in procedure. Once properly silanated, the ceramic surface becomes hydrophobic, and the try-in paste can be easily removed by ultrasonic cleansing. Current scientific evidences[20] show that if the try-in step is done after silanation, bond strengths will increase significantly. This can be explained by the fact that the try-in procedure removes the excessive layers of silane from ceramic surface.[20] The removal of excess permits proper coupling of the resin cement with the monolayer-silanated ceramic surface, thus improving the bond strength. Moreover, silane treatment alone seems to be very effective to improve bond strengths to ceramic. Thus, when the try-in step is involved, it should rather be done after silanation, followed by ultrasonic cleanse for better bond strength.

A durable bond with high-strength polycrystalline ceramic systems has been proved to be a difficult task. The use of a silane-coupling agent after airborne particle abrasion

(APA) did not result in a durable resin bond to zirconium.[75,76] As an alternative, silicoating has been proposed to create an additional silica layer over the reinforced ceramic cores to allow for bonding procedures. However, some reports demonstrated a significant reduction in the bond strength after simulated artificial aging in zirconium-based ceramics treated with silicoating followed by silanization.[75,77,78] Reinforced ceramic core systems are not as dependent on bonding as the fragile feldspathic ceramics. Manufacturers' recommendations for luting reinforced ceramic cores suggest the use of conventional cements such as zinc phosphate or resin-modified glass ionomer. However, adhesive cementation has been shown to increase its fracture resistance and longevity[79,80]; sealing of internal surface flaws created by airborne particle abrasion (APA)[81]; and working as auxiliary retention to its inherent loose fit.

Many different chemo-mechanical surface treatments have demonstrated effectiveness in optimizing the cement/reinforced ceramic bonding interface.[82–84] Slight differences in the sintering temperature may influence the final poly-crystal structure, grain sizes, and mechanical properties. Thus, different ceramics reactions to specific surface treatments may be expected.[82] Several studies have investigated if these treatments, combined or not, can promote more durable bonds to reinforced ceramic cores. Among them, there is airborne particle abrasion (APA) or wet hand grinding, use of phosphate ester and phosphoric acid monomers present either in resin luting cements or some primers; tribochemical silicoating, laser irradiation, selective infiltration–etching (SIE) technique by heat treatment, and others. To date, however, there is no clinical consensus regarding the best surface conditioning method for achieving optimum bond strength to reinforced ceramics. Despite these invaluable efforts, the clinical significance of bonding to high-strength ceramics and its influence on the long-term survival warrants future investigation.

APA APA or wet hand grinding is an alternative widely investigated for improved resin bonding to reinforced ceramics.[83] Some research groups have demonstrated that these mechanical surface modifications significantly increased the flexural strength of Yttria-stabilized tetragonal zirconia polycrystal (Y-TZP)[83,85–87] by inducing a tetragonal to monolithic phase transformation that could inhibit microcrack extension, thus increasing the strength of zirconium. Conversely, other scientific evidences are showing that surface treatments such as grinding or sandblasting Y-TZP ceramics before cementation may create surface defects and sharp cracks that can be stress concentration sources that render the zirconium framework susceptible to radial cracking during function.[88,89] Significantly lower reliability for zirconium core ceramics was demonstrated for two postsintered cementation surface modification techniques, grinding and alumina abrasion, when compared with the as-received zirconium cores.[90] In 2005, Guazzato and colleagues[85] detected a significant amount of monoclinic phase (9.5%) after sandblasting but no monoclinic phase detection after heat treatment. Authors assumed that the compressive stresses created were released, and the mean flexural strength obtained was related to the defects induced by sandblasting without the benefits of the transformed region. Thus, they assumed that any temporary beneficial effect induced by different surface treatment methods could be counteracted by fatigue-related crack growth phenomena.[85]

Low-pressure air abrasion (0.05 MPa) was proposed as an alternative to improve bond strength[91,92] without compromising the ceramic structure. The authors of both studies stated that although the surface roughness was reduced, it did not affect the long-term bond strength. However, omitting air abrasion resulted in debonding during artificial aging, independent of using primers.[91] In 2010, Aboushelib and colleagues[93] demonstrated that APA specimens may have their flexural strength recovered by the application of the bonding agent. Standard error of the mean analysis of the fractured surfaces indicated that application of the bonding agent resulted in sealing of the surface damage produced by APA. Additionally, Casucci and colleagues[82] (2010) evaluated the surface roughness for three different ceramics and a significant increase in the average surface roughness of Cercon (DETREY DENTSPLY) (DeguDent, Hanau, Germany) and Aadva (GC Corporation, Tokyo, Japan) Zr ceramics were found, while no differences were produced on Lava (3M ESPE, St Paul, MN, USA). Thus, manufacturers' recommendations must be taken under consideration regarding APA and wet grinding mechanical surface modification, because ceramics perform differently in response to the same APA approach.

Resin cements and primers containing 10-MDP monomer (10-methacryloyloxydecyl dihydrogenphosphate) have been considered the materials of choice because of the chemical interaction established between the hydroxyl groups of the zirconia ceramic and the phosphate ester monomer of the MDP-containing material.[94,95] Resin luting cements as Panavia,[96] and some primers as Alloy Primer, Clearfil Ceramic Primer (Kuraray, Osaka, Japan) are representatives of this type of material. The use of zirconia 10-MDP-based primers in combination with APA improved resin bond strength, immediately and in long-term evaluations.[78,83,91,97,98] However, more recently, Aboushelib and colleagues[93] observed bond strength reduction after artificial aging for the APA group in combination with application of MDP monomer. Authors[93] related the contradiction to the fact that their study used microbars instead of discs, which expose more surface area of the bonded interface to the influence of water. Primers containing phosphoric acid monomer as Metal/Zirconia Primer (Ivoclar-Vivadent) and AZ Primer (Shofu) are also considered alternative to promote the adhesion to oxide ceramics such as zirconia and alumina, because they are claimed to achieve chemical bond to the oxidic ceramic surface.[91,97] Differences in chemical composition of the primers and their bonding mechanisms require adequate combination of surface treatments and the proper selection of primer according to each commercial resin cement system.[98] In general, primers containing a phosphonic acid monomer or phosphate ester monomer improve resin bonding to zirconia ceramics, while primers containing a silane-coupling agent improve resin bonding to silica–base ceramics.[97] A new zirconia experimental primer, based on a mixture of organophosphate and carboxylic acid monomers, has been recently investigated as another alternative to increase bond strength of different resin-based luting agents.[99]

Tribochemical silicoating Tribochemical silicoating has been claimed as an alternative to APA, in an attempt to improve the bond between alumina/zirconia ceramics and resin cements.[100] In this technique, the surfaces are airborne-particle abraded with aluminum trioxide particles modified with silica. The blasting pressure results in the embedding of the silica-coated alumina particles on the ceramic surface, rendering the silica-modified surface chemically reactive to the resin through silane-coupling agents. Some studies have demonstrated high bond strength values of resin to zirconia after silicoating and silanation.[83,101] However, when artificial aging was proposed, it resulted in significant decrease in bond strengths of resin to silicoated zirconia.[76–78] The authors further indicated that thermal cycling had a greater impact on the durability of the resin bond to zirconia ceramic than water storage at constant temperature.[76–78]

New approaches to enhance bonds to high-strength polycrystalline ceramics A newly developed surface treatment has been proposed to improve zirconia bonding, the selective infiltration etching (SIE) technique by heat treatment.[93] It transforms the zirconia from a dense, nonretentive, and low-energy surface to a highly active and retentive surface. In this procedure, the surface is coated with a glass-containing conditioning agent (composed of silica, alumina, sodium oxide potassium oxide, and titanium oxide) and heated above its glass transition temperature. After cooling, the glass is dissolved in an acidic bath, creating a porous surface and achieving promising results in terms of bond strength to resin cements. In 2010, Aboushelib and colleagues[93] demonstrated that SIE established a strong, stable, and durable bond to zirconia substrates as well. Stanard error of the mean analysis demonstrated that the surface topography created a highly retentive surface where the adhesive resin penetrated and interlocked. Even though the depth of resin tags was limited to 0.3 μm to 0.7μm, the porosities allowed for the establishment of a strong nanomechanical bond with the adhesive resin used, which resisted nanoleakage during artificial aging.[93]

Alternatively, laser irradiation has been introduced as another treatment option for zirconia and alumina surfaces. Er,Cr:YSGG laser should be considered an innovative alternative for promoting adhesion of ceramics (glass-infiltrated alumina) to resin cement, since it resulted in similar bond strength values compared with the tribochemical treatment.[102] Also, CO_2 laser etching may represent an effective method for conditioning zirconia surfaces, enhancing micromechanical retention, and improving the bond strength of resin cement on zirconia ceramic.[84]

SUMMARY

Clinical trials are required to understand what the real performance of new ceramics in the oral environment may be and what the role of luting agents and surface treatments on their performance may be. In addition, many other individual factors are involved in a clinical failure, such as core design and thickness and damage by processing and handling, added to the occlusal function. The high number of clinical complications with all-ceramic fixed dental prostheses, even with increased connector size,[103] requires clinical attention in the material selection, and an important improvement of the veneering system is still required.[104] Up to date, there are a limited number of published clinical trials on Y-TZP and other reinforced core ceramics, but it has the potential for being accepted as a suitable material for fixed prosthodontics.[105]

In addition, it is important to evaluate the long-term performance of different surface treatments. Other approaches are expected to be developed to improve/stabilize the bonding mechanisms to teeth and all-ceramic systems involving, for instance, chemical function of the tooth and ceramic substrates via increase of the amount of –OH groups and consequently the wet ability response on the surfaces prior bonding, potentially enhancing the long-term expectation of ceramic/cement/substrate interface.

ACKNOWLEDGMENTS

The authors thank Dr Van Thompson, chair of the department of Biomaterials and Biomimetics at New York University College of Dentistry for his guidance and editorial support.

REFERENCES

1. Meyer JM, Cattani-Lorente MA, Dupuis V. Compomers: between glass–ionomer cements and composites. Biomaterials 1998;19(6):529–39.
2. Rosenstiel SF, Land MF, Crispin BJ. Dental luting agents: a review of the current literature. J Prosthet Dent 1998;80(3):280–301.
3. O'Brien W. Dental materials and their selection. 3rd edition. Chicago (IL): Quintessence; 2002. p. 133–55.

4. Wettstein F, Sailer I, Roos M, et al. Clinical study of the internal gaps of zirconia and metal frameworks for fixed partial dentures. Eur J Oral Sci 2008;116(3):272–9.

5. Yiu CK, Tay FR, King NM, et al. Interaction of glass–ionomer cements with moist dentin. J Dent Res 2004;83(4):283–9.

6. Glasspoole EA, Erickson RL, Davidson CL. Effect of surface treatments on the bond strength of glass ionomers to enamel. Dent Mater 2002;8:454–62.

7. Naasan MA, Watson TF. Conventional glass ionomers as posterior restorations. A status report for the American Journal of Dentistry. Am J Dent 1998;11(1): 36–45.

8. Kerby RE, Knobloch L. Strength characteristics of glass–ionomer cements. Oper Dent 1992;17(5):170–4.

9. Peumans M, Van Meerbeek B, Lambrechts P, et al. Porcelain veneers: a review of the literature. J Dent 2000;28(3):163–77.

10. Christensen GJ. The rise of resin for cementing restorations. J Am Dent Assoc 1993;124(10):104–5.

11. Breeding LC, Dixon DL, Caughman WF. The curing potential of light-activated composite resin luting agents. J Prosthet Dent 1991;65(4):512–8.

12. Caughman WF, Chan DC, Rueggeberg FA. Curing potential of dual-polymerizable resin cements in simulated clinical situations. J Prosthet Dent 2001;86(1):101–6.

13. Myers ML, Caughman WF, Rueggeberg FA. Effect of restoration composition, shade, and thickness on the cure of a photoactivated resin cement. J Prosthodont 1994;3(3):149–57.

14. Anusavice KJ. Phillips' science of dental materials. 11th edition. Philadelphia: Saunders Elsevier; 2003.

15. Mitra SB. Dental cements: formulations and handling techniques. In: Curtis VR, Watson T, editors. Dental biomaterials. Imaging, testing, and modeling. Boca Raton (FL): Woodhead Publishing Limited and CRC Press LLC; 2008. p. 27.

16. el-Badrawy WA, el-Mowafy OM. Chemical versus dual curing of resin inlay cements. J Prosthet Dent 1995;73(6):515–24.

17. Hasegawa EA, Boyer DB, Chan DC. Hardening of dual-cured cements under composite resin inlays. J Prosthet Dent 1991;66(2):187–92.

18. Pereira SG, Fulgencio R, Nunes TG, et al. Effect of curing protocol on the polymerization of dual-cured resin cements. Dent Mater 2010;26(7):710–8.

19. Pegoraro TA. Efeito do protocolo de ativação da polimerização e envelhecimento acelerado em algumas propriedades de cimentos resinosos. Bauru (Brazil): Reabilitação Oral, Faculdade de Odontologia de Bauru, Universidade de São Paulo; 2010 [in Portuguese].

20. Pegoraro TA, da Silva NR, Carvalho RM. Cements for use in esthetic dentistry. Dent Clin North Am 2007;51(2):453–71.

21. Peutzfeldt A, Asmussen E. Investigations on polymer structure of dental resinous materials. Trans Acad Dent Mater 2004;18:81–104.

22. Carvalho RM, Garcia FC, e Silva SM, et al. Adhesive–composite incompatibility, part II. J Esthet Restor Dent 2005;17(3):191–5.

23. Tay FR, Pashley DH, Yiu CK, et al. Factors contributing to the incompatibility between simplified-step adhesives and chemically cured or dual-cured composites. Part I. Single-step self-etching adhesive. J Adhes Dent 2003; 5(1):27–40.

24. Tay FR, Suh BI, Pashley DH, et al. Factors contributing to the incompatibility between simplified-step adhesives and self-cured or dual-cured composites. Part II. Single-bottle, total-etch adhesive. J Adhes Dent 2003;5(2):91–105.

25. Cheong C, King NM, Pashley DH, et al. Incompatibility of self-etch adhesives with chemical/dual-cured composites: two-step vs one-step systems. Oper Dent 2003;28(6):747–55.
26. Sanares AM, Itthagarun A, King NM, et al. Adverse surface interactions between one-bottle light-cured adhesives and chemical-cured composites. Dent Mater 2001;17(6):542–56.
27. Suh BI, Feng L, Pashley DH, et al. Factors contributing to the incompatibility between simplified-step adhesives and chemically cured or dual-cured composites. Part III. Effect of acidic resin monomers. J Adhes Dent 2003;5(4):267–82.
28. Carvalho RM, Pegoraro TA, Tay FR, et al. Adhesive permeability affects coupling of resin cements that utilise self-etching primers to dentine. J Dent 2004;32(1): 55–65.
29. Tay FR, Pashley DH, Suh BI, et al. Single-step adhesives are permeable membranes. J Dent 2002;30:371–82.
30. King NM, Tay FR, Pashley DH, et al. Conversion of one-step to two-step self-etch adhesives for improved efficacy and extended application. Am J Dent 2005; 18(2):126–34.
31. Cury AH, Goracci C, de Lima Navarro MF, et al. Effect of hygroscopic expansion on the push-out resistance of glass ionomer-based cements used for the luting of glass fiber posts. J Endod 2006;32(6):537–40.
32. Goracci C, Fabianelli A, Sadek FT, et al. The contribution of friction to the dislocation resistance of bonded fiber posts. J Endod 2005;31(8):608–12.
33. Paul SJ, Scharer P. The dual bonding technique: a modified method to improve adhesive luting procedures. Int J Periodontics Restorative Dent 1997;17(6): 536–45.
34. Duarte S Jr, de Freitas CR, Saad JR, et al. The effect of immediate dentin sealing on the marginal adaptation and bond strengths of total-etch and self-etch adhesives. J Prosthet Dent 2009;102(1):1–9.
35. Hu J, Zhu Q. Effect of immediate dentin sealing on preventive treatment for post-cementation hypersensitivity. Int J Prosthodont 2010;23(1):49–52.
36. Duke ES. New technology directions in resin cements. Compend Contin Educ Dent 2003;24(8). 606–8, 610.
37. Burke FJ, Crisp RJ, Richter B. A practice based evaluation of the handling of a new self-adhesive universal resin luting material. Int Dent J 2006;56(3): 142–6.
38. Radovic I, Monticelli F, Goracci C, et al. Self-adhesive resin cements: a literature review. J Adhes Dent 2008;10(4):251–8.
39. De Munck J, Van Landuyt K, Peumans M, et al. A critical review of the durability of adhesion to tooth tissue: methods and results. J Dent Res 2005;84(2):118–32.
40. Gerth HU, Dammaschke T, Zuchner H, et al. Chemical analysis and bonding reaction of RelyX Unicem and Bifix composites—a comparative study. Dent Mater 2006;22(10):934–41.
41. Abo-Hamar SE, Hiller KA, Jung H, et al. Bond strength of a new universal self-adhesive resin luting cement to dentin and enamel. Clin Oral Investig 2005;9(3): 161–7.
42. Hikita K, Van Meerbeek B, De Munck J, et al. Bonding effectiveness of adhesive luting agents to enamel and dentin. Dent Mater 2007;23(1):71–80.
43. De Munck J, Vargas M, Van Landuyt K, et al. Bonding of an autoadhesive luting material to enamel and dentin. Dent Mater 2004;20(10):963–71.
44. Al-Assaf K, Chakmakchi M, Palaghias G, et al. Interfacial characteristics of adhesive luting resins and composites with dentine. Dent Mater 2007;23(7):829–39.

45. Flury S, Lussi A, Peutzfeldt A, et al. Push-out bond strength of CAD/CAM-ceramic luted to dentin with self-adhesive resin cements. Dent Mater 2010; 26(9):855–63.
46. Guarda GB, Goncalves LS, Correr AB, et al. Luting glass ceramic restorations using a self-adhesive resin cement under different dentin conditions. J Appl Oral Sci 2010;18(3):244–8.
47. Tanoue N, Koishi Y, Atsuta M, et al. Properties of dual-curable luting composites polymerized with single and dual curing modes. J Oral Rehabil 2003;30(10): 1015–21.
48. Fan PL, Edahl A, Leung RL, et al. Alternative interpretations of water sorption values of composite resins. J Dent Res 1985;64(1):78–80.
49. Ortengren U, Elgh U, Spasenoska V, et al. Water sorption and flexural properties of a composite resin cement. Int J Prosthodont 2000;13(2):141–7.
50. Oysaed H, Ruyter IE. Composites for use in posterior teeth: mechanical properties tested under dry and wet conditions. J Biomed Mater Res 1986;20(2): 261–71.
51. Ferracane JL, Berge HX, Condon JR. In vitro aging of dental composites in water—effect of degree of conversion, filler volume, and filler/matrix coupling. J Biomed Mater Res 1998;42(3):465–72.
52. Huang M, Niu X, Shrotriya P, et al. Contact damage of dental multilayers: viscous deformation and fatigue mechanisms. J Eng Mater Technol 2005;127(33):33–9.
53. Braden M, Clarke RL. Water absorption characteristics of dental microfine composite filling materials. I. Proprietary materials. Biomaterials 1984;5(6): 369–72.
54. Pearson GJ, Longman CM. Water sorption and solubility of resin-based materials following inadequate polymerization by a visible-light curing system. J Oral Rehabil 1989;16(1):57–61.
55. Vrochari AD, Eliades G, Hellwig E, et al. Water sorption and solubility of four self-etching, self-adhesive resin luting agents. J Adhes Dent 2010;12(1):39–43.
56. Scherrer SS, de Rijk WG, Belser UC, et al. Effect of cement film thickness on the fracture resistance of a machinable glass–ceramic. Dent Mater 1994;10(3): 172–7.
57. Magne P, Kwon KR, Belser UC, et al. Crack propensity of porcelain laminate veneers: a simulated operatory evaluation. J Prosthet Dent 1999;81(3):327–34.
58. Silva NR, de Souza GM, Coelho PG, et al. Effect of water storage time and composite cement thickness on fatigue of a glass–ceramic trilayer system. J Biomed Mater Res B Appl Biomater 2008;84(1):117–23.
59. Cekic-Nagas I, Canay S, Sahin E. Bonding of resin core materials to lithium disilicate ceramics: the effect of resin cement film thickness. Int J Prosthodont 2010;23(5):469–71.
60. Van Noort R. Introduction to dental materials. 3rd edition. London: Mosby Elsevier; 2007.
61. Raigrodski AJ, Chiche GJ. All-ceramic fixed partial dentures. Part I: in vitro studies. J Esthet Restor Dent 2002;14(3):188–91.
62. Raigrodski AJ, Chiche GJ, Potiket N, et al. The efficacy of posterior three-unit zirconium-oxide-based ceramic fixed partial dental prostheses: a prospective clinical pilot study. J Prosthet Dent 2006;96(4):237–44.
63. Raigrodski AJ, Chiche GJ, Swift EJ Jr. All-ceramic fixed partial dentures. Part III: clinical studies. J Esthet Restor Dent 2002;14(5):313–9.
64. Sailer I, Feher A, Filser F, et al. Five-year clinical results of zirconia frameworks for posterior fixed partial dentures. Int J Prosthodont 2007;20(4):383–8.

65. Sailer I, Philipp A, Zembic A, et al. A systematic review of the performance of ceramic and metal implant abutments supporting fixed implant reconstructions. Clin Oral Implants Res 2009;20(Suppl 4):4–31.

66. Sailer I, Pjetursson BE, Zwahlen M, et al. A systematic review of the survival and complication rates of all-ceramic and metal–ceramic reconstructions after an observation period of at least 3 years. Part II: fixed dental prostheses. Clin Oral Implants Res 2007;18(Suppl 3):86–96.

67. Tinschert J, Schulze KA, Natt G, et al. Clinical behavior of zirconia-based fixed partial dentures made of DC-Zirkon: 3-year results. Int J Prosthodont 2008; 21(3):217–22.

68. Clelland NL, Warchol N, Kerby RE, et al. Influence of interface surface conditions on indentation failure of simulated bonded ceramic onlays. Dent Mater 2006;22(2):99–106.

69. Blatz MB, Sadan A, Kern M. Resin–ceramic bonding: a review of the literature. J Prosthet Dent 2003;89(3):268–74.

70. Barghi N, Chung K, Farshchian F, et al. Effects of the solvents on bond strength of resin-bonded porcelain. J Oral Rehabil 1999;26(11):853–7.

71. Hooshmand T, van Noort R, Keshvad A. Bond durability of the resin-bonded and silane-treated ceramic surface. Dent Mater 2002;18(2):179–88.

72. Meng XF, Yoshida K, Gu N. Chemical adhesion rather than mechanical retention enhances resin bond durability of a dental glass–ceramic with leucite crystallites. Biomed Mater 2010;5(4):044101.

73. Ishida H. Structural gradient in the silane-coupling agent layers and its influence on the mechanical and physical properties of composites. New York (NY): Plenum Press; 1985. p. 25–50.

74. Hooshmand T, van Noort R, Keshvad A. Storage effect of a preactivated silane on the resin to ceramic bond. Dent Mater 2004;20(7):635–42.

75. Derand T, Molin M, Kvam K. Bond strength of composite luting cement to zirconia ceramic surfaces. Dent Mater 2005;21(12):1158–62.

76. Kern M, Wegner SM. Bonding to zirconia ceramic: adhesion methods and their durability. Dent Mater 1998;14(1):64–71.

77. Ozcan M, Vallittu PK. Effect of surface conditioning methods on the bond strength of luting cement to ceramics. Dent Mater 2003;19(8):725–31.

78. Wegner SM, Kern M. Long-term resin bond strength to zirconia ceramic. J Adhes Dent 2000;2(2):139–47.

79. Della Bona A, Kelly JR. The clinical success of all-ceramic restorations. J Am Dent Assoc 2008;139:8S–13S.

80. Scherrer SS, De Rijk WG, Belser UC. Fracture resistance of human enamel and three all-ceramic crown systems on extracted teeth. Int J Prosthodont 1996;9(6): 580–5.

81. Blatz MB. Long-term clinical success of all-ceramic posterior restorations. Quintessence Int 2002;33(6):415–26.

82. Casucci A, Mazzitelli C, Monticelli F, et al. Morphological analysis of three zirconium oxide ceramics: effect of surface treatments. Dent Mater 2010;26(8): 751–60.

83. Qeblawi DM, Munoz CA, Brewer JD, et al. The effect of zirconia surface treatment on flexural strength and shear bond strength to a resin cement. J Prosthet Dent 2010;103(4):210–20.

84. Ural XC, Külünk T, Külünk S, et al. Determination of resin bond strength to zirconia ceramic surface using different primers. Acta Odontol Scand 2010; 69:48–53.

85. Guazzato M, Quach L, Albakry M, et al. Influence of surface and heat treatments on the flexural strength of Y-TZP dental ceramic. J Dent 2005;33(1):9–18.

86. Kosmac T, Oblak C, Jevnikar P, et al. The effect of surface grinding and sand-blasting on flexural strength and reliability of Y-TZP zirconia ceramic. Dent Mater 1999;15(6):426–33.

87. Kosmac T, Oblak C, Jevnikar P, et al. Strength and reliability of surface treated Y-TZP dental ceramics. J Biomed Mater Res 2000;53(4):304–13.

88. Lawn BR, Deng Y, Lloyd IK, et al. Materials design of ceramic-based layer struc-tures for crowns. J Dent Res 2002;81(6):433–8.

89. Zhang Y, Lawn BR, Rekow ED, et al. Effect of sandblasting on the long-term performance of dental ceramics. J Biomed Mater Res B Appl Biomater 2004; 71(2):381–6.

90. Guess PC, Zhang Y, Kim JW, et al. Damage and reliability of Y-TZP after cemen-tation surface treatment. J Dent Res 2010;89(6):592–6.

91. Kern M, Barloi A, Yang B. Surface conditioning influences zirconia ceramic bonding. J Dent Res 2009;88(9):817–22.

92. Yang B, Barloi A, Kern M. Influence of air-abrasion on zirconia ceramic bonding using an adhesive composite resin. Dent Mater 2010;26(1):44–50.

93. Aboushelib MN, Feilzer AJ, Kleverlaan CJ. Bonding to zirconia using a new surface treatment. J Prosthodont 2010;19(5):340–6.

94. Oyague RC, Monticelli F, Toledano M, et al. Effect of water aging on microtensile bond strength of dual-cured resin cements to pretreated sintered zirconium-oxide ceramics. Dent Mater 2009;25(3):392–9.

95. Tanaka R, Fujishima A, Shibata Y, et al. Cooperation of phosphate monomer and silica modification on zirconia. J Dent Res 2008;87(7):666–70.

96. Blatz MB, Sadan A, Martin J, et al. In vitro evaluation of shear bond strengths of resin to densely sintered high-purity zirconium oxide ceramic after long-term storage and thermal cycling. J Prosthet Dent 2004;91(4):356–62.

97. Kitayama S, Nikaido T, Takahashi R, et al. Effect of primer treatment on bonding of resin cements to zirconia ceramic. Dent Mater 2010;26(5):426–32.

98. Yun JY, Ha SR, Lee JB, et al. Effect of sandblasting and various metal primers on the shear bond strength of resin cement to Y-TZP ceramic. Dent Mater 2010; 26(7):650–8.

99. Magne P, Paranhos MP, Burnett LH Jr. New zirconia primer improves bond strength of resin-based cements. Dent Mater 2010;26(4):345–52.

100. Kern M, Thompson VP. Sandblasting and silica coating of a glass-infiltrated alumina ceramic: volume loss, morphology, and changes in the surface compo-sition. J Prosthet Dent 1994;71(5):453–61.

101. Kim BK, Bae HE, Shim JS, et al. The influence of ceramic surface treatments on the tensile bond strength of composite resin to all-ceramic coping materials. J Prosthet Dent 2005;94(4):357–62.

102. de Paula Eduardo C, Bello-Silva MS, Moretto SG, et al. Microtensile bond strength of composite resin to glass-infiltrated alumina composite conditioned with Er, Cr:YSGG laser. Lasers Med Sci 2010. [Epub ahead of print].

103. Land MF, Hopp CD. Survival rates of all-ceramic systems differ by clinical indi-cation and fabrication method. J Evid Based Dent Pract 2010;10(1):37–8.

104. Schley JS, Heussen N, Reich S, et al. Survival probability of zirconia-based fixed dental prostheses up to 5 yr: a systematic review of the literature. Eur J Oral Sci 2010;118(5):443–50.

105. Al-Amleh B, Lyons K, Swain M. Clinical trials in zirconia: a systematic review. J Oral Rehabil 2010;37(8):641–52.

All-Ceramic Systems: Laboratory and Clinical Performance

Petra C. Guess, DDS, Dr Med Dent[a],*, Stefan Schultheis, DDS, Dr Med Dent[a],
Estevam A. Bonfante, DDS, MSc, PhD[b], Paulo G. Coelho, DDS, PhD[c],
Jonathan L. Ferencz, DDS[d], Nelson R.F.A. Silva, DDS, MSc, PhD[d]

KEYWORDS

• All-ceramic material • CAM/CAD • Zirconia • Alumina

Over the last 3 decades, a trend to shift toward metal-free restorations has been observed in the dental field. To meet the increased demands of patients and dentists for highly aesthetic, biocompatible, and long-lasting restorations, several types of all-ceramic systems have been developed.[1] Silicate and glass ceramics are used as a veneer for metal or all-ceramic cores to optimize form and aesthetics. In a monolithic application, small-sized restorations such as inlays, onlays, laminate veneers, and crowns can also be fabricated. High-strength ceramics such as aluminum and zirconium oxide ceramics were developed as a core material for crowns and fixed dental prostheses (FDPs) to extend the indication ranges to the high-load bearing areas.[2] Most recently, monolithic zirconia restorations are increasingly promoted for single-crown and full-mouth rehabilitation, in particular for patients with parafunctional habits.

Because of advances in computer aided design (CAD) and computer aided manufacturing (CAM) technologies, the high-strength ceramic systems have become increasingly popular. Zirconia, specifically yttria-containing tetragonal zirconia polycrystal (Y-TZP), with unsurpassed mechanical properties (**Table 1**), has had its clinical application expanded from single crowns and short-span FDPs to multiunit and full-arch zirconia frameworks as well as to implant abutments and complex implant superstructures to support fixed and removable prostheses.[3,4] Zirconia in its pristine form can be considered as a reliable framework material with reported failure rates lower

[a] Department of Prosthodontics, Dental School, Albert-Ludwigs University, Hugstetter Street 55, 79106 Freiburg, Germany
[b] Department of Prosthodontics, UNIGRANRIO University, School of Dentistry, Rio de Janeiro, Brazil
[c] Department of Biomaterials and Biomimetics, New York University College of Dentistry, New York, NY, USA
[d] Department of Prosthodontics, New York University College of Dentistry, New York, NY, USA
* Corresponding author.
E-mail address: petra.guess@uniklinik-freiburg.de

Dent Clin N Am 55 (2011) 333–352
doi:10.1016/j.cden.2011.01.005
0011-8532/11/$ – see front matter © 2011 Elsevier Inc. All rights reserved.

Table 1
Mechanical properties of different all-ceramic systems according to manufacturer's instructions

Material	Modulus (GPa)	Hardness (GPa)	Toughness (MPa m$^{1/2}$)	Strength (MPa)	CTE°C X × 10^{-6}	Firing (°C)
Porcelain						
Vitablocks (feldspathic)	45	NA	NA	154	9.4	780–790
Lava Ceram	78	5.3	1.1	100	10.5	810
IPS e.max ceram	60–70	5.4	NA	90	9.5	750
IPS e.max ZirPress (flour-apatite)	65	5.4	NA	110	10.5–11	900–910
Glass-ceramic						
Dicor	75	3.4	1.4	290	9.8	850
Empress esthetic (leucite)	65–68	6.2	1.3	160	16.6–17.5	625
IPS e.max Press (lithium disilicate)	95	5.8	2.75	400	10.2–10.5	915–920
IPS e.max CAD (lithium disilicate)	95	5.8	2.25	360	10.2–10.5	840
Alumina						
In-Ceram Alumina	280	20	3.5	500	7.2	2053 melting point
Procera Alumina	340	17	3.2	695	7.0	1600
Zirconia						
Cercon	210	12	9	1300	10.5	1350
IPS e.max Zir CAD	210	13	5.5	900	10.8	1500
Lava	210	14	5.9	1048	10.5	1480
DSC Zirkon	210	12	7	1200	10.4	1500
In-Ceram YZ	210	12	5.9	>900	10.5	2706 melting point
Procera Zirconia	210	14	6	1200	10.4	1550
Prettau Zirkon Zirkonzahn	210	12.5	NA	1000	10	1600
Tooth						
Dentin	16	0.6	3.1	—	11–14	—
Enamel	94	3.2	0.3	—	2–8	—

Abbreviations: CTE, coefficient of thermal expansion; NA, not available.

than those observed for silicate or alumina frameworks (**Table 2**).[5] However, questions regarding the overall success of bilayer zirconia/veneer restorations have been raised as a result of early chipping/fracture events observed[6] while in oral function. As a result, various research groups have tried to better understand the potential problems such as the thermal interaction between the ceramic core and veneering porcelain, their respective processing techniques, and the effect of framework configuration on veneer support, in an attempt to overcome early chippings/fractures and enhance the long-term service of all-ceramic systems.

This overview presents the current knowledge of monolithic and bilayer all-ceramic systems and addresses composition and processing mechanisms, laboratory and clinical performance, and possible future trends.

REINFORCED GLASS CERAMICS

The interest in nonmetallic and biocompatible restorative materials increased after the introduction of the feldspathic porcelain crown in 1903 by Land.[7] In 1965, McLean[8] pioneered the concept of adding aluminum oxide to feldspathic porcelain in an attempt to enhance mechanical properties. However, the clinical shortcomings of these materials, such as brittleness, crack propagation, low tensile strength, wear resistance, and marginal accuracy, discontinued its use.[9]

Increased strength in glassy ceramics can be achieved by adding appropriate fillers that are uniformly dispersed throughout the glass, a technique termed dispersion strengthening. Leucite is used as a reinforcing crystalline at a concentration of 35 to 45 vol%.[10] In the early 1990s, the lost wax press technique was introduced to dentistry as an innovative processing method for all-ceramic restorations. Examples of leucite-reinforced glass ceramics are VITA VMK 68 (VITA Zahnfabrik, Bad Säckingen, Germany), Finesse All-Ceramic, (Dentsply, York, PA, USA), Optec OPC (Jeneric, Wallingford, CT, USA), and IPS Empress (Ivoclar Vivadent, Schaan, Principality of Liechtenstein). The molding procedure of IPS Empress is conducted at 1080°C in a special, automatically controlled furnace. Leucite crystals are formed through a controlled surface crystallization process in the SiO_2-Al_2O_3-K_2O glass system. Tangential compressive stresses develop around the crystals on cooling because of the difference in the coefficient of thermal expansion (CTE) between leucite crystals and the glassy matrix. These stresses contribute to crack deflection and improved mechanical performance.[11] IPS Empress, for instance, exhibits a flexural strength of 120 to 180 MPa and a CTE of 15 to 18.5×10^{-6} K^{-1} m/m.[12] The material is suitable for fabrication of inlays, onlays, veneers, and crowns. Favorable clinical long-term data with high survival rates are described for IPS Empress inlays, onlays (90% after 8 years[13]), veneers (94.4% after 12 years[14]), and crowns (95.2% after 11 years[15]) in the dental literature.

Leucite glass ceramics can also be machined with various CAD/CAM systems. Multi-colored blocks were recently developed to reproduce color transitions and shading as well as different levels of translucency to reproduce natural teeth (**Fig. 1**).[16] The use of leucite-reinforced glass ceramic has significantly declined because of the introduction of lithium disilicate glass ceramics with significantly improved mechanical and aesthetic properties and is addressed in detail in the next section.

LITHIUM DISILICATE GLASS CERAMICS

A significantly higher strength of 350 MPa was achieved with a glass ceramic of the SiO_2-Li_2O-K_2O-ZnO-P_2O_5-Al_2O_3-La_2O_3 system by precipitating lithium disilicate ($Li_2Si_2O_5$) crystals. The crystal content of up to 70 vol% is considerably higher than that of leucite materials.[11] High-temperature x-ray diffraction studies revealed that both lithium metasilicate (Li_2SiO_3) and crystobalite form during the crystallization process before the growth of lithium disilicate ($Li_2Si_2O_5$) crystals.[17] The final microstructure consists of highly interlocked lithium disilicate crystals, 5 μm in length and 0.8 μm in diameter. Thermal expansion mismatch between lithium disilicate crystals and glassy matrix results in tangential compressive stresses around the crystals, potentially responsible for crack deflection and strength increase. Crystal alignment after heat pressing of the lithium disilicate glass ceramic leads to multiple crack

Table 2
Clinical outcomes of zirconia-based crowns and FDPs

Study	Ceramic Materials	Observation Period (y)	Type of Restoration	Sample Size	Survival Rate (%)	Framework Fracture (%)	Veneer Fracture (%)
Cehreli et al,[61] 2009	Cercon Veneer n.s.	2	Single crowns	15	NS	7	0
Groten & Huttig,[108] 2010	Cercon Cercon Ceram Kiss	2	Single crowns	54	98	0	9
Ortorp et al,[68] 2009	Noble Procera Zirconia Vita Lumin Noble Rondo Zirconia	3	Single crowns	204	92.7	0	2
Schmitt et al,[109] 2010	Lava Lava Ceram	3	Single crowns	19	100	0	5
Schmitter et al,[67] 2009	Cercon Cercon Ceram S	2	4- to 7-unit FDP	30	96.6	3	3
Tsumita et al,[110] 2010	Cercon Creation ZI	2	3-unit FDP	21	NS	0	14
Sailer et al,[69] 2009	Cercon Cercon Ceram S	3	3- to 5-unit FDP	38	100	0	25
Beuer et al,[63] 2009	Cercon Cercon Ceram Express	3	3-unit FDP	21	90.5	5	0
Roediger et al,[64] 2010	Cercon Cercon Ceram S Experimental veneering ceramic	4	3- to 4-unit FDP	99	94	1	13
Wolfart et al,[75] 2009	Cercon Cercon Ceram S Cercon Ceram Express	4	3- to 4-unit FDP/Cantilever FDP	24 34	96 92	0 0	13 12

Sailer et al,[62] 2007	Cercon Experimental veneering ceramic	3- to 5-unit FDP	5	57	73.9	8	15
Crisp et al,[111] 2008	Lava Lava Ceram	3- to 4-unit FDP	1	38	100	0	3
Raigrodski et al,[112] 2006	Lava Veneer n.s.	3-unit FDP	2.5	20	NS	0	25
Schmitt et al,[113] 2009	Lava Lava Ceram	3- to 4-unit FDP	3	27	100	0	11
Vult von Steyern et al,[114] 2005	DC Zirkon Vita D	3- to 5-unit FDP	2	20	NS	0	15
Tinschert et al,[83] 2008	DC Zirkon Vita D	3- to 10-unit FDP/Cantilever FDP	3	65	NS	0	6
Edelhoff et al,[115] 2008	Digident Initial ZirKeramik GC	3- to 6-unit FDP	3	21	90.5	0	10
Molin and Karlsson,[116] 2008	Denzir Vita D IPS Empress	3-unit FDP	5	19	100	0	36
Nothdurft & Pospiech,[84] 2009	Cercon Cercon Ceram Kiss	Implant-supported single crowns	0.5	40	NS	0	8
Larsson et al,[49] 2006	Denzir Esprident Triceram	Implant-supported FDP	1	13	NS	0	53
Larsson et al,[3] 2010	Cercon Cercon Ceram S	Implant-supported full-arch FDP	3	10	100	0	34

Abbreviation: NS, not specified.

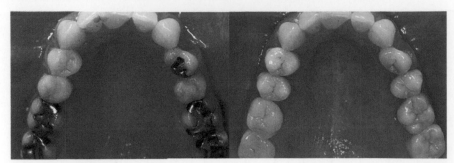

Fig. 1. Before and after treatment with all-ceramic restorations (lithium disilicate IPS e.max Press Tooth 24 inlay; onlays 26, 27; and crowns14, 15, 25) and CAD/CAM-fabricated leucite ProCAD onlay 16, 26.

deflections. The lithium disilicate ceramic was introduced as IPS Empress 2 (Ivoclar Vivadent) in 1998 and is moldable as leucite glass ceramics, but at a lower temperature of 920°C. The CTE is 10.5×10^{-6} K^{-1} m/m.[18]

High survival rates were observed for anterior and posterior IPS Empress 2 crowns (95.5% after 10 years[19]) in long-term clinical studies (**Fig. 2**). The clinical success of 3-unit IPS Empress 2 FDPs is predominately limited by bulk fracture failure within the connector area, in particular when the connector size is less than the recommended dimensions (70% survival rate after 5 years[20]) (**Fig. 3**).

A newly developed pressable lithium disilicate glass ceramic (IPS e.max Press, Ivoclar Vivadent) with improved physical properties (flexural strength, 440 MPa) and translucency through different firing process has been developed in the SiO_2-Li_2O-K_2O-ZnO-P_2O_5-Al_2O_3-ZrO_2 system. The pressable lithium disilicate ceramic can be used in monolithic application for inlays, onlays, and posterior crowns or as a core material for crowns and 3-unit FDPs in the anterior region. Apatite glass ceramics are recommended for veneering.

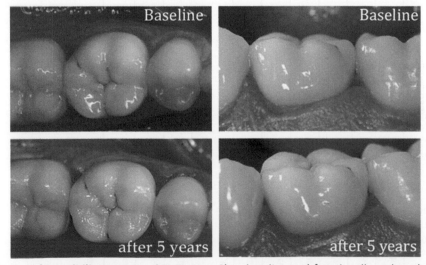

Fig. 2. Lithium disilicate crowns (IPS Empress 2) at baseline and functionally and aesthetically successful performance after 5 years.

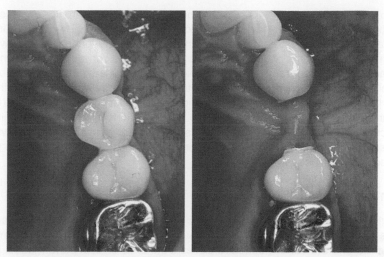

Fig. 3. Three-unit lithium disilicate (IPS Empress 2) FDPs at baseline and a connector bulk fracture after 11 months.

Clinical data exhibited high survival rates on IPS e.max Press onlays (100% after 3 years),[21] crowns (96,6% after 3 years),[22] monolithic inlay retained FDPs (100% after 4 years),[23] and full crown retained FDPs (93% after 8 years).[24]

Recently, a lithium disilicate glass ceramic (IPS e.max CAD, Ivoclar Vivadent) has been designed for CAD/CAM processing technology. The milled lithium disilicate block is exposed to a 2-stage crystallization process. Lithium metasilicate crystals are precipitated during the first stage. The resulting glass ceramic has a crystal size range of 0.2 to 1.0 μm with approximately 40 vol% lithium metasilicate crystals. At this pre-crystallized state, the CAD/CAM block exhibits a flexural strength of 130 to 150 MPa, which allows simplified machining and intraoral occlusal adjustment. The final crystal-lization process occurs after milling of the restoration at 850°C in vacuum. The meta-silicate crystal phase is dissolved completely, and the lithium disilicate crystallizes. This process also converts the blue shade of the precrystallized block to the selected tooth shade and results in a glass ceramic with a fine grain size of approximately 1.5 μm and a 70% crystal volume incorporated in a glass matrix.[16] CAD/CAM-processed lithium disilicate glass ceramic demonstrates a flexural strength of 360 MPa (see **Table 1**). Because of the favorable translucency and shade assortment the material can be used for fully anatomic (monolithic) restorations with subsequent staining char-acterization or as a core material with subsequent coating with veneering ceramics. The manufacturer recommends its use for anterior or posterior crowns, implant crowns, inlays, onlays, and veneers. Preliminary clinical results on single crowns revealed high survival rates (100% after 2 years[25]) and are hence extremely promising.

GLASS-INFILTRATED CERAMICS

Another group of all-ceramic systems involves glass-infiltrated ceramics. In-Ceram Alumina (VITA Zahnfabrik) was the first all-ceramic system available for single-unit restorations and 3-unit anterior bridges[26] with a high-strength ceramic core fabricated with the slip-casting technique.[27] A slurry of densely packed (70–80 wt%) Al_2O_3 is applied and sintered to a refractory die at 1120°C for 10 hours.[28,29] This process produces a porous skeleton of alumina particles, which is infiltrated with lanthanum glass in a second firing at 1100°C for 4 hours to eliminate porosity and increase strength.[29] The core is veneered with feldspathic porcelain.[26] In-Ceram Zirconia (VITA Zahnfabrik) is a modification of the original In-Ceram Alumina system, with an addition of 35% partially stabilized zirconia oxide to the slip composition to strengthen the ceramic.[27] Traditional slip-casting techniques can be used, or the material can be copy-milled from prefabricated, partially sintered blanks and then veneered with feldspathic porcelain.[30] As the core is opaque and lacks translucency, the use of this material for anterior regions becomes problematic.[27] Clinical performance of glass-infiltrated ceramics for crowns and FDPs indication has been evaluated in a systematic review.[31] However, with the development of high-strength ceramics, recent literature on glass-infiltrated ceramics became sparse.

HIGH-STRENGTH OXIDE CERAMICS

Although high-strength ceramic in dentistry includes alumina and zirconia, this section focuses mainly on zirconia because of its superior mechanical properties compared with alumina and the current controversial aspects of its clinical performance.

Zirconia ceramics have gained a remarkable interest in biomedical sciences.[4] The first reference concerning their application in medicine appeared in the late sixties; 20 years later, Christel and colleagues[32] studied their use in orthopedic surgery.[33] In the early 1990s, zirconia was introduced to dentistry,[34] and in recent years, a large number of publications appeared in the literature.

Zirconia, characterized by a dense, monocrystalline homogeneity, possesses low thermal conductivity, low corrosion potential, and good radiopacity.[4] High biocompatibility, low bacterial surface adhesion, and favorable optical properties of zirconia ceramics are reported.[35–37] Zirconia in its pure form is a polymorph that has 3 temperature-dependant phases that are monoclinic (room temperature to 1170°C), tetragonal (1170°C–2370°C), and cubic (2370°C to melting point).[34] With the addition of stabilizing oxides such as magnesia, ceria, yttria, and calcium to zirconia, the tetragonal phase is retained in a metastable condition at room temperature, enabling a phenomenon called transformation toughening to occur. In response to mechanical stimuli, the partially stabilized crystalline tetragonal zirconia transforms to the more-stable monoclinic phase, with a local volume increase of approximately 4%. This increase in volume counteracts further crack propagation by compression at the tip of the crack.[38] Compared with high-strength alumina ceramic, zirconia has twice the flexural strength (900–1200 MPa).[39,40] In addition, high fracture toughness (9–10 $MPa \cdot m^{1/2}$) has been described.[39] The most commonly used dental zirconia formulations are glass-infiltrated zirconia toughened alumina ceramics (In-Ceram, VITA Zahnfabrik) and 3 mol% Y-TZP. Y-TZP has been used for root canal posts,[41] frameworks for posterior teeth, implant-supported crowns, multiunit FDPs,[42] resin-bonded FDPs,[43] custom-made bars to support fixed and removable dental prostheses,[44] implant abutments,[45,46] and dental implants.[47,48]

A magnesium-doped partially stabilized zirconia (Mg-PSZ, Denzir M, Dentronic AB, Sweden) is available, but porosity and large grain size has limited its success.[49]

Zirconia and CAD/CAM Technology

An array of CAD/CAM systems has evolved since F. Duret introduced the concept in 1971.[50,51] Some CAD/CAM systems (Denzir, Cadesthetics, Skellefteå, Sweden, and DC-Zircon, DCS Dental AG, Allschwil, Switzerland) machine fully sintered Y-TZP blocks, which have been processed by hot isostatic pressing. Because of the hardness and poor machinability of fully sintered Y-TZP, a robust milling system and extended milling periods are required. Most of the available CAD/CAM systems shape blocks of partially sintered zirconia.[34] Milling from partially sintered blocks involves machining enlarged frameworks in a so-called green state. These blocks are then sintered to their full strength, which is accompanied by shrinkage of the milled framework by approximately 25% to the desired dimensions. Examples of these systems are CERCON (Dentsply Friadent, Mannheim, Germany), LAVA (3M ESPE, Seefeld, Germany), Procera (Nobel Biocare, Gothenburg, Sweden), Etkon (Straumann, Basel, Switzerland), and Cerec (Sirona, Bensheim, Germany).

The advantage of industrialized blank fabrication and reproducible and consistent CAM resulted in increased process reliability and cost-effectiveness of CAD/CAM-fabricated restorations.[52] Labor-intensive waxing, casting, and soldering of frameworks accompanied with conventional laboratory procedures can be avoided with the application of CAD/CAM technology. With extensive frameworks, particularly used in implant dentistry, and the escalating costs of precious alloys, all-ceramic restorations are competitive with conventional metal-ceramic restorations (MCRs) from a cost perspective.[53]

Zirconia and Low-Temperature Degradation

A major drawback of zirconia restorations compared with metal-ceramics is the material-inherent accelerated aging that has been observed to occur in zirconia in the presence of moisture.[54,55] This aging phenomenon is known as low-temperature degradation (LTD) and was first described by Kobayashi and colleagues[56] in 1981. At relatively low temperatures (150°C–400°C), slow tetragonal to monoclinic transformations occur, initiating at the surface of polycrystalline zirconia and subsequently progressing into the bulk of the material.[34,57] Transformation of 1 grain is accompanied by an increase in volume, which causes stress on the surrounding grains and microcracking. Water penetration into these cracks then exacerbates the process of surface degradation, and the transformation progresses. The growth of the transformation zone results in severe microcracking, grain pullout, and finally surface roughening, which ultimately leads to strength degradation. Any factor that is detrimental to the stability of tetragonal zirconia is susceptible to promote LTD. Among these factors are grain size,[58] the amount of stabilizer,[59] and the presence of residual stress.[54,60] At present, there is no clear correlation between LTD and failure predictability when zirconia is used as a dental bioceramic.[33]

Clinical Data on Zirconia-Supported Restorations

Although zirconia was introduced to dentistry in the early 1990s, limited information about its clinical performance can be found. A literature search from 1990 through September 2010 using electronic databases (PubMed and MEDLINE) revealed a total of 21 clinical trials on zirconia-supported restorations (see **Table 2**). Long-term clinical data for zirconia-supported restorations with observation periods exceeding 5-year time frames are not yet available. Most studies (n = 14) investigated predominately posterior FDPs, whereas a small number focused on (n = 4) crowns. Only 3 studies described the clinical behavior of implant-supported zirconia-supported FDPs and single crowns.

Veneered Zirconia Clinical Failure Modes

Core/framework fractures

Catastrophic fractures within the zirconia core ceramic are reported at 7% for single crowns after 2 years and at 1% to 8% for FDPs after 2 to 5 years (see **Table 2**). Occlusal overloading caused by bruxism (crown fracture after 1 month[61]) or trauma (connector fracture 5-unit FDP after 38 months[62]) and insufficient framework thickness at 0.3 mm (crown-abutment fractures in 3-unit FDP[63,64]) were mentioned as the main reasons for zirconia core bulk fractures. Fractographic analyses of clinically failed zirconia crowns showed that radial fractures propagating upwards from the cementation surface site resulted in bulk fractures and caused catastrophic failures of the restorations.[65] Microscopic examinations of failed zirconia-based FDPs revealed that core bulk fractures were most commonly located in the connector area and initiated from the gingival surface, where tensile stresses were the greatest because of occlusal loading.[65,66] Core bulk fracture in the connector area was also attributed to damage induced during fabrication.[67] A higher susceptibility to connector fracture was noted with an increased span of FDPs.[65]

Veneering ceramic cohesive fractures
The major drawbacks noted in all clinical studies on zirconia-supported restorations were less related to the framework integrity than to wear and failure of the veneering ceramics. Cohesive fractures within the veneering ceramic (chipping) were described as the most frequent reason for failures, irrespective of the applied zirconia veneer system (see **Table 2**). Veneer fracture rates are reported at 2% to 9% for single crowns after 2 to 3 years and at 3% to 36% for FDPs after 1 to 5 years. Implant-supported zirconia-based restorations revealed even higher rates at 8% for single crowns after 6 months and at 53% for FDPs after 1 year. Impaired proprioception and rigidity of osseointegrated implants correlated with higher functional impact forces might further exacerbate cohesive veneer fractures. To date, only one 3-year prospective clinical study involving implant-supported full-arch Y-TZP reconstructions is available. Despite the short follow-up period and limited number of patients (n = 10), no framework fractures were observed; however, chip-off fractures were observed in 34% of the units cemented in 9 of 10 patients.[3]

Depending on the size and localization, cracks leading to veneer fractures can severely compromise the aesthetics and function of zirconia-supported restorations.[68,69] Fractographic analysis of clinically failed veneered zirconia restorations revealed cohesive veneer failures, with cracks originating from the occlusal surface and propagating to the core veneer interface, leaving an intact core.[65] In many clinical studies, it seemed that these veneer failures were associated with roughness in the veneering ceramic because of occlusal function or occlusal adjustment.[49,69,70] Therefore, special attention has to be paid to the static and dynamic aspects of occlusion in zirconia-based restorations. Occlusal adjustments should be performed only with fine-grain diamonds under water irrigation followed by a thorough polishing sequence.

Reasons for veneering ceramic failure
As the veneering ceramic material (flexural strength, approximately 90–120 MPa) is weak compared with the high-strength core material (900–1200 MPa),[39,40] the veneering ceramic seems to be prone to failure at low loads during masticatory function. The use of higher-strength veneering ceramic was proposed to reduce the incidence of veneer chippings/fractures. However, attempts to improve the microstructure and mechanical properties of veneering ceramics with the development of glass-ceramic ingots for pressing veneering ceramics onto zirconia frameworks did not result in an increased reliability of the veneering ceramic.[71,72] In addition, identical chip-failure patterns were observed.[71–74] Although a high density of the veneering layer has been expected with the press technique, spherical porosities were noted within the veneer layer and also at the interface.[72] In clinical trials on zirconia FDPs, chipping fractures have also been reported with pressable veneering ceramics, and the chipping problem does not seem to be solved.[75]

Moreover, the CTE is frequently discussed as a contributing factor for veneer failure. However, the problem of chipping may not be limited only to the mismatch of CTE; it seems more complex. Residual stresses in bilayer crowns and FDPs are associated with the possibility of thermal gradients being developed in these structures during cooling. For zirconia veneer all-ceramic systems, the low thermal conductivity of the zirconia (approximately 3 Wm/K)[76] results in the highest temperature difference and, therefore, very high residual stresses. In addition, thick layers of veneering ceramics on zirconia cores are highly susceptible to generating high tensile subsurface residual stresses, ultimately resulting in unstable cracking or chipping.[77] Slow cooling of the restoration above the glass transition temperature of the porcelain could prevent the development of high tensile subsurface residual stresses in the porcelain, which may result in unstable cracking or chipping. Most manufacturers now recommend the approach of a reduced cooling rate after final firing or glazing, and even an additional 6 minutes has shown to be effective.[78]

Zirconia framework design

The lack of a uniform support of the veneering ceramic because of improper framework design has been discussed as a possible reason for chipping fractures. Remarkably little scientific clinical data on optimal design of zirconia-supported restorations have been published.[53,79,80] With the introduction of CAD/CAM technologies in dentistry, excessive veneer layer thickness (>2.5 mm) was created because of the uniform layer thickness of the copings for crowns and bar-shaped connectors for FDPs. Improved customized zirconia coping design derived from the conventional porcelain fused to metal technique has been recommended to provide adequate support for the veneering ceramic.[80] A dual-scan procedure of the die and full-contour wax pattern has been merged to fabricate the desired framework. Preliminary in vitro studies showed that cohesive fractures within the veneering ceramic could not be avoided with the improved support, but the size of the fractures was significantly decreased[81,82] and failure initiation was shifted toward higher loads.[73] In clinical observation, conflicting results on the framework design modification have been described.[83,84] Hence, the effect of framework design modifications on residual stress states needs to be better elucidated.[77]

Minimizing Zirconia Core Failures

Some fundamental aspects affecting the clinical performance of zirconia as a framework material need to be addressed. Laboratory technicians and clinicians should follow the precise sequence steps in manufacturing zirconia-based restorations, with the knowledge that zirconia as a framework material is potentially damaged by surface modifications and improper laboratory and clinical handling techniques.[85]

Grinding or sandblasting of surfaces with high (or mild/low) pressure ranges is implicated as a factor in inducing the formation of surface microcracking[85-87] that could be detrimental to the long-term performance of the restorations and lead to unexpected failures.[88] Several research groups have claimed an increased flexural strength in Y-TZP[89] because of phase transformation after grinding and alumina abrasion.[90-92] However, any temporary beneficial effect related to phase transformation induced by different surface treatment methods may be negated by fatigue-related crack growth phenomena and following heat treatments associated with veneer application.[90] With respect to the highly deleterious effect on zirconia reliability,[93] postsintering surface modifications of zirconia frameworks at the dental laboratory or under clinical circumstances should be avoided.

LABORATORY PERFORMANCE OF ALL-CERAMIC MATERIALS

Randomized prospective clinical trials are the first choice for evaluating clinical long-term behavior of dental materials and techniques. However, the results of clinical investigations are restricted by high costs, and meaningful conclusions can be drawn only if an adequate number of restorations are incorporated and observed for at least 3 to 4 years.[94] In addition, fractures are occasionally observed after 4 to 5 years of clinical service (Ferencz J, personal communication, 2010). Therefore, in vitro simulations and laboratory tests are developed to investigate new dental materials and predict lifetimes and failures.

Various testing methods have been used to investigate the mechanical properties of dental materials. Many concerns have been raised lately regarding the clinical significance of simple traditional mechanical testing methodologies and single load to failure tests of dental restorations, loosely termed "crunch the crown test"[95] or flexural strength tests. These tests report unrealistically high fracture strength values, largely overestimating the actual failure load. Furthermore, the obtained failure modes differ significantly from those reported in clinical observations. Hence, little insight into damage initiation and propagation can be provided.[96] In material science, fatigue is the progressive and localized structural damage that occurs when a material is subjected to cyclic loading. Fatigue is a significant factor limiting the lifespan of zirconia-based restorations and, therefore, represents a prerequisite for valid in vitro testing.[97] A recently developed mouth-motion fatigue model has demonstrated the ability to duplicate clinical fractures[98] and predict the material's reliability to validate its clinical potential.

Guess and colleagues[99] examined the failure and fatigue behavior of a hand-layer veneered zirconia core ceramic and compared it with a monolithic CAD/CAM-fabricated lithium disilicate ceramic. A sliding contact mouth-motion fatigue testing in water on anatomically correct crowns was applied to simulate approximating tooth surfaces during mastication. Hand-layer veneered zirconia crowns supported by tooth replicas revealed a high single-cycle load to failure strength of 1195 ± 221 N. But during mouth-motion fatigue testing, hand-layer veneered zirconia-based crowns resulted in a very limited reliability; approximately 90% of specimens failed from veneer chip-off fracture by 100,000 cycles at 200 N. Failure progressed from the contact area through the body of the veneering ceramic as noted in clinical cases.[65] The observed fatigue behavior of zirconia-supported crowns does not seem to be material or system dependent, as similar results were reported in previous findings using the identical test methodology.[100] In contrast, CAD/CAM lithium disilicate crowns showed no failures up to load levels exceeding posterior physiologic chewing forces and seemed to be resistant to mouth-motion step-stress (900 N/180,000 cycles) and also to staircase fatigue (1000 N/1 million cycles).[101] A threshold for damage and bulk fracture could be detected in the range of 1100 to 1200 N. CAD/CAM processing of the lithium disilicate ceramic uses industrialized fabricated homogenous ceramic blanks; therefore, the material reveals a high density with a minimum of inherent flaws. Increased Weibull modulus and reliability have been reported for CAD/CAM-fabricated materials.[102] Conversely, the presence of structural "impurities" within the veneer layer of zirconia-supported ceramics is a known drawback of bilayer all-ceramic systems.[71]

The Gold-Standard Metal-Ceramic

Although MCRs are frequently referred to as the gold standard and still represent a common procedure to rehabilitate missing dental structures and teeth, limited information is available regarding their clinical and laboratory performance when compared with all-ceramic systems. After the introduction of zirconia to dentistry, more elaborate clinical and laboratory investigations were performed, but MCRs were, in most instances, not included as control.[103,104] Moreover, the understanding of the failure mechanisms of MCRs is mainly related to biological issues rather than fracture or chipping of the veneer porcelain.[105]

In one of the few laboratory studies presented in the dental literature, Silva and colleagues[74] performed a sliding contact fatigue test study on anatomically correct MCR crowns and compared the reliability and failure modes with zirconia-supported crowns. **Fig. 4** shows a series of representative images of laboratory-tested MCRs, zirconia-supported crowns, and its clinical-matched fractures. The resemblance of failure modes for both systems shows the potential of use sliding

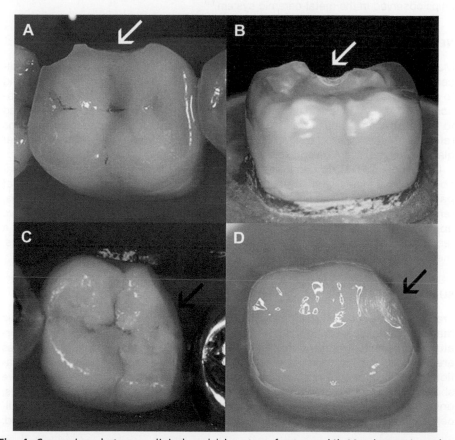

Fig. 4. Comparison between clinical and laboratory fractures. (A) Metal-ceramic molar crown fractured after about 13 years of oral function. (B) Representative metal-ceramic molar crown after step-stress mouth-motion fatigue test. White arrows in (A) and (B) show typical veneer cohesive fractures. (C) Typical clinical veneer cohesive fracture (*black arrow*) at the proximal aspect of a Y-TZP-supported all-ceramic crown after 2.5 years in oral function. (D) Typical fracture (*black arrow*) at the proximal aspect of a Y-TZP-supported all-ceramic crown after a mouth-motion fatigue test. Note similar fracture pattern compared with clinical failure mode shown in (C). ([A] *Courtesy of* Dr Carlo Marinello, University of Basel, Switzerland.)

contact fatigue concept to preclinical scenarios. The investigators[74] observed that the MCR system presented a significantly higher reliability compared with Y-TZP, which may explain the fact that not many reports of veneer fractures for MCRs can be found. As new ceramic systems, including more robust monolithic materials, are available in the market, it becomes imperative that further laboratory and clinical investigations including MCR as control are needed. To date, only 1 randomized controlled clinical trial involving 3- to 5-unit zirconia-supported fixed partial dentures has been performed with metal-ceramic as controls. The findings of this 3-year follow-up have shown no differences among biological or technical complications between the 2 systems. Chip-off fractures occurred in 25% of the zirconia-supported prostheses and in 19.4% of the metal-ceramics. Although the chipping occurrence was not statistically different between the groups, only the zirconia-supported prostheses presented unacceptable major fractures of the veneering ceramic relative to the minor chips observed in the metal-ceramic system.[69]

NEW CONCEPTS FOR THE ALL-CERAMIC SYSTEMS

Many manufacturers have shifted their attention to the development of monolithic all-ceramic materials to simply remove the most common failing layer of the system and to avoid inherent residual thermal stresses in bilayer all-ceramic systems. In combination with CAD/CAM fabrication, monolithic/full-anatomic crown restorations seemed to be reliable and robust. Most recently, monolithic zirconia ceramic restorations refined with superficial glazing and staining and functionally graded glass/zirconia/glass structures[106] are being explored in high-load bearing areas.

In addition, CAD/CAM capabilities creating separate core and veneer layers that could then be joined with nonthermal methods will continue to evolve and are of particular interest for extended restorations.[107] Subtractive CAD/CAM approaches, removing material from a block to create a shape, will be complemented by additive approaches, depositing materials only in places where it is needed to form a restoration.[74] Although issues are still remaining with each of these approaches, they show great promise.

SUMMARY

Fracture of the veneering ceramics, thermal interaction between core and ceramic materials, and susceptibility of zirconia to aging are still being debated in the dental literature. Refinement of framework design and innovative CAD/CAM veneering techniques are promising tools to improve the clinical performance of zirconia-supported restorations. The use of monolithic leucite and lithium disilicate glass ceramic systems have shown promising laboratory and clinical results for small restorations such as inlays, onlays, crowns, and laminates. Further laboratory and clinical investigations using all-ceramic materials compared with metal-ceramic systems are strongly recommended.

ACKNOWLEDGMENTS

The authors thank the Department of Biomaterials and Biomimetics at the New York University College of Dentistry, USA. The authors also thank Dr Leonard Marotta (Marotta Dental Studios) for substantial collaboration. Special acknowledgment to Drs Van P. Thompson, Elizabeth Dianne Rekow and Joerg R. Strub for their support and professional guidance.

REFERENCES

1. Denry I, Holloway JA. Ceramics for dental applications: a review. Materials 2010;3:351–68.
2. Conrad HJ, Seong WJ, Pesun IJ. Current ceramic materials and systems with clinical recommendations: a systematic review. J Prosthet Dent 2007;98(5): 389–404.
3. Larsson C, Vult von Steyern P, Nilner K. A prospective study of implant-supported full-arch yttria-stabilized tetragonal zirconia polycrystal mandibular fixed dental prostheses: three-year results. Int J Prosthodont 2010;23(4):364–9.
4. Manicone PF, Rossi Iommetti P, Raffaelli L. An overview of zirconia ceramics: basic properties and clinical applications. J Dent 2007;35(11):819–26.
5. Della Bona A, Kelly JR. The clinical success of all-ceramic restorations. J Am Dent Assoc 2008;139(Suppl):8S–13S.
6. Al-Amleh B, Lyons K, Swain M. Clinical trials in zirconia: a systematic review. J Oral Rehabil 2010;37(8):641–52.
7. Land CH. Porcelain dental art. Dental Cosmos 1903;45:437–615.
8. McLean JW, Hughes TH. The reinforcement of dental porcelain with ceramic oxides. Br Dent J 1965;119:251–67.
9. Sjögren G, Lantto R, Granberg A, et al. Clinical examination of leucite-reinforced glass-ceramic crowns (Empress) in general practice: a retrospective study. Int J Prosthodont 1999;12(2):122–8.
10. Denry I, Rosenstiel SF. Phase tranformation in feldspathic dental porcelains. In: Fischman G, editor. Bioceramics: materials and applications. Westervill (OH): The American Ceramic Society; 1995.
11. Guazzato M, Albakry M, Ringer SP, et al. Strength, fracture toughness and microstructure of a selection of all-ceramic materials. Part I. Pressable and alumina glass-infiltrated ceramics. Dent Mater 2004;20(5):441–8.
12. Dong JK, Luthy H, Wohlwend A, et al. Heat-pressed ceramics: technology and strength. Int J Prosthodont 1992;5(1):9–16.
13. Kramer N, Taschner M, Lohbauer U, et al. Totally bonded ceramic inlays and onlays after eight years. J Adhes Dent 2008;10(4):307–14.
14. Fradeani M, Redemagni M, Corrado M. Porcelain laminate veneers: 6- to 12-year clinical evaluation–a retrospective study. Int J Periodontics Restorative Dent 2005;25(1):9–17.
15. Fradeani M, Redemagni M. An 11-year clinical evaluation of leucite-reinforced glass-ceramic crowns: a retrospective study. Quintessence Int 2002;33(7): 503–10.
16. Höland W, Schweiger M, Watzke R, et al. Ceramics as biomaterials for dental restoration. Expert Rev Med Devices 2008;5(6):729–45.
17. Höland W, Apel E, vańt Hoen C, et al. Studies of crystal phase formation in the early stage crystallization of lithium disilicate glass-ceramics. J Non Cryst Solids 2006;352:4041–50.
18. Höland W, Schweiger M, Frank M, et al. A comparison of the microstructure and properties of the IPS Empress 2 and the IPS Empress glass-ceramics. J Biomed Mater Res 2000;53(4):297–303.
19. Valenti M, Valenti A. Retrospective survival analysis of 261 lithium disilicate crowns in a private general practice. Quintessence Int 2009;40(7):573–9.
20. Marquardt P, Strub JR. Survival rates of IPS empress 2 all-ceramic crowns and fixed partial dentures: results of a 5-year prospective clinical study. Quintessence Int 2006;37(4):253–9.

21. Guess PC, Strub JR, Steinhart N, et al. All-ceramic partial coverage restorations–midterm results of a 5-year prospective clinical splitmouth study. J Dent 2009;37(8):627–37.

22. Etman MK, Woolford MJ. Three-year clinical evaluation of two ceramic crown systems: a preliminary study. J Prosthet Dent 2010;103(2):80–90.

23. Wolfart S, Bohlsen F, Wegner SM, et al. A preliminary prospective evaluation of all-ceramic crown-retained and inlay-retained fixed partial dentures. Int J Prosthodont 2005;18(6):497–505.

24. Wolfart S, Eschbach S, Scherrer S, et al. Clinical outcome of three-unit lithium-disilicate glass-ceramic fixed dental prostheses: up to 8 years results. Dent Mater 2009;25(9):e63–e71.

25. Fasbinder DJ, Dennison JB, Heys D, et al. A clinical evaluation of chairside lithium disilicate CAD/CAM crowns: a two-year report. J Am Dent Assoc 2010; 141(Suppl 2):10S–4S.

26. Haselton DR, Diaz-Arnold AM, Hillis SL. Clinical assessment of high-strength all-ceramic crowns. J Prosthet Dent 2000;83(4):396–401.

27. Sundh A, Sjogren G. A comparison of fracture strength of yttrium-oxide-partially-stabilized zirconia ceramic crowns with varying core thickness, shapes and veneer ceramics. J Oral Rehabil 2004;31(7):682–8.

28. Chai J, Takahashi Y, Sulaiman F, et al. Probability of fracture of all-ceramic crowns. Int J Prosthodont 2000;13(5):420–4.

29. Xiao-ping L, Jie-mo T, Yun-long Z, et al. Strength and fracture toughness of MgO-modified glass infiltrated alumina for CAD/CAM. Dent Mater 2002;18(3): 216–20.

30. Raigrodski AJ. Contemporary materials and technologies for all-ceramic fixed partial dentures: a review of the literature. J Prosthet Dent 2004;92(6):557–62.

31. Wassermann A, Kaiser M, Strub JR. Clinical long-term results of VITA In-Ceram Classic crowns and fixed partial dentures: a systematic literature review. Int J Prosthodont 2006;19(4):355–63.

32. Christel P, Meunier A, Dorlot JM, et al. Biomechanical compatibility and design of ceramic implants for orthopedic surgery. Ann N Y Acad Sci 1988;523:234–56.

33. Chevalier J. What future for zirconia as a biomaterial? Biomaterials 2006;27(4): 535–43.

34. Denry I, Kelly JR. State of the art of zirconia for dental applications. Dent Mater 2008;24(3):299–307.

35. Aboushelib MN, Dozic A, Liem JK. Influence of framework color and layering technique on the final color of zirconia veneered restorations. Quintessence Int 2010;41(5):e84–e89.

36. Degidi M, Artese L, Scarano A, et al. Inflammatory infiltrate, microvessel density, nitric oxide synthase expression, vascular endothelial growth factor expression, and proliferative activity in peri-implant soft tissues around titanium and zirconium oxide healing caps. J Periodontol 2006;77(1):73–80.

37. Rimondini L, Cerroni L, Carrassi A, et al. Bacterial colonization of zirconia ceramic surfaces: an in vitro and in vivo study. Int J Oral Maxillofac Implants 2002;17(6):793–8.

38. Garvie RC, Hannink RH, Pascoe RT. Ceramic steel? Nature 1975;258:703–4.

39. Christel P, Meunier A, Heller M, et al. Mechanical properties and short-term in-vivo evaluation of yttrium-oxide-partially-stabilized zirconia. J Biomed Mater Res 1989;23(1):45–61.

40. Piconi C, Maccauro G. Zirconia as a ceramic biomaterial. Biomaterials 1999; 20(1):1–25.

41. Meyenberg KH, Luthy H, Scharer P. Zirconia posts: a new all-ceramic concept for nonvital abutment teeth. J Esthet Dent 1995;7(2):73–80.
42. Sturzenegger B, Fehér A, Luthy H, et al. Clinical evaluation of zirconium oxide bridges in the posterior segments fabricated with the DCM system. Acta Med Dent Helv 2000;5:131–9.
43. Komine F, Tomic M. A single-retainer zirconium dioxide ceramic resin-bonded fixed partial denture for single tooth replacement: a clinical report. J Oral Sci 2005;47(3):139–42.
44. Bergler M, Holst S, Blatz MB, et al. CAD/CAM and telescopic technology: design options for implant-supported overdentures. Eur J Esthet Dent 2008; 3(1):66–88.
45. Glauser R, Sailer I, Wohlwend A, et al. Experimental zirconia abutments for implant-supported single-tooth restorations in esthetically demanding regions: 4-year results of a prospective clinical study. Int J Prosthodont 2004;17(3): 285–90.
46. Sailer I, Philipp A, Zembic A, et al. A systematic review of the performance of ceramic and metal implant abutments supporting fixed implant reconstructions. Clin Oral Implants Res 2009;20(Suppl 4):4–31.
47. Andreiotelli M, Wenz HJ, Kohal RJ. Are ceramic implants a viable alternative to titanium implants? A systematic literature review. Clin Oral Implants Res 2009; 20(Suppl 4):32–47.
48. Wenz HJ, Bartsch J, Wolfart S, et al. Osseointegration and clinical success of zirconia dental implants: a systematic review. Int J Prosthodont 2008;21(1):27–36.
49. Larsson C, Vult von Steyern P, Sunzel B, et al. All-ceramic two- to five-unit implant-supported reconstructions. A randomized, prospective clinical trial. Swed Dent J 2006;30(2):45–53.
50. Miyazaki T, Hotta Y, Kunii J, et al. A review of dental CAD/CAM: current status and future perspectives from 20 years of experience. Dent Mater J 2009; 28(1):44–56.
51. Rekow ED. Dental CAD/CAM systems: a 20-year success story. J Am Dent Assoc 2006;137(Suppl):5S–6S.
52. Tinschert J, Natt G, Hassenpflug S, et al. Status of current CAD/CAM technology in dental medicine. Int J Comput Dent 2004;7(1):25–45.
53. Donovan TE. Factors essential for successful all-ceramic restorations. J Am Dent Assoc 2008;139(Suppl):14S–8S.
54. Deville S, Chevalier J, Gremillard L. Influence of surface finish and residual stresses on the ageing sensitivity of biomedical grade zirconia. Biomaterials 2006;27(10):2186–92.
55. Tholey MJ, Berthold C, Swain MV, et al. XRD(2) micro-diffraction analysis of the interface between Y-TZP and veneering porcelain: role of application methods. Dent Mater 2010;26(6):545–52.
56. Kobayashi K, Kuwajima H, Masaki T. Phase change and mechanical properties of ZrO2-Y2O3 solid electrolyte after aging. Solid State Ionics 1981;3:489–93.
57. Kelly JR, Denry I. Stabilized zirconia as a structural ceramic: an overview. Dent Mater 2008;24(3):289–98.
58. Lawson S. Environmental degradation of zirconia ceramics. J Eur Ceram Soc 1995;15:485–502.
59. Hannink R, Kelly PM, Muddle B. Transformation toughening in zirconia containing ceramics. J Am Ceram Soc 2000;83(3):461–87.
60. Kim JW, Covel NS, Guess PC, et al. Concerns of hydrothermal degradation in CAD/CAM zirconia. J Dent Res 2010;89(1):91–5.

61. Cehreli MC, Kokat AM, Akca K. CAD/CAM Zirconia vs. slip-cast glass-infiltrated Alumina/Zirconia all-ceramic crowns: 2-year results of a randomized controlled clinical trial. J Appl Oral Sci 2009;17(1):49–55.
62. Sailer I, Feher A, Filser F, et al. Five-year clinical results of zirconia frameworks for posterior fixed partial dentures. Int J Prosthodont 2007;20(4):383–8.
63. Beuer F, Edelhoff D, Gernet W, et al. Three-year clinical prospective evaluation of zirconia-based posterior fixed dental prostheses (FDPs). Clin Oral Investig 2009;13(4):445–51.
64. Roediger M, Gersdorff N, Huels A, et al. Prospective evaluation of zirconia posterior fixed partial dentures: four-year clinical results. Int J Prosthodont 2010;23(2):141–8.
65. Aboushelib MN, Feilzer AJ, Kleverlaan CJ. Bridging the gap between clinical failure and laboratory fracture strength tests using a fractographic approach. Dent Mater 2009;25(3):383–91.
66. Taskonak B, Yan J, Mecholsky JJ Jr, et al. Fractographic analyses of zirconia-based fixed partial dentures. Dent Mater 2008;24(8):1077–82.
67. Schmitter M, Mussotter K, Rammelsberg P, et al. Clinical performance of extended zirconia frameworks for fixed dental prostheses: two-year results. J Oral Rehabil 2009;36(8):610–5.
68. Ortorp A, Kihl ML, Carlsson GE. A 3-year retrospective and clinical follow-up study of zirconia single crowns performed in a private practice. J Dent 2009; 37(9):731–6.
69. Sailer I, Gottnerb J, Kanelb S, et al. Randomized controlled clinical trial of zirconia-ceramic and metal-ceramic posterior fixed dental prostheses: a 3-year Follow-up. Int J Prosthodont 2009;22(6):553–60.
70. Hobkirk JA, Wiskott HW. Ceramics in implant dentistry (Working Group 1). Clin Oral Implants Res 2009;20(Suppl 4):55–7.
71. Tsalouchou E, Cattell MJ, Knowles JC, et al. Fatigue and fracture properties of yttria partially stabilized zirconia crown systems. Dent Mater 2007;24(3):308–18.
72. Guess PC, Zhang Y, Thompson VP. Effect of veneering techniques on damage and reliability of Y-TZP trilayers. Eur J Esthet Dent 2009;4(3):262–76.
73. Bonfante EA, Rafferty B, Zavanelli RA, et al. Thermal/mechanical simulation and laboratory fatigue testing of an alternative yttria tetragonal zirconia polycrystal core-veneer all-ceramic layered crown design. Eur J Oral Sci 2010;118(2): 202–9.
74. Silva NR, Bonfante EA, Zavanelli RA, et al. Reliability of metalloceramic and zirconia-based ceramic crowns. J Dent Res 2010;89(10):1051–6.
75. Wolfart S, Harder S, Eschbach S, et al. Four-year clinical results of fixed dental prostheses with zirconia substructures (Cercon): end abutments vs. cantilever design. Eur J Oral Sci 2009;117(6):741–9.
76. Birkby I, Stevens R. Applications of zirconia ceramics. Key Eng Mater 1996; 122–124:527–52.
77. Swain MV. Unstable cracking (chipping) of veneering porcelain on all-ceramic dental crowns and fixed partial dentures. Acta Biomater 2009;5(5):1668–77.
78. Rues S, Kroger E, Muller D, et al. Effect of firing protocols on cohesive failure of all-ceramic crowns. J Dent 2010;38:987–94.
79. Pogoncheff CM, Duff RE. Use of zirconia collar to prevent interproximal porcelain fracture: a clinical report. J Prosthet Dent 2010;104(2):77–9.
80. Marchack B, Futatsuki Y, Marchack C, et al. Customization of milled zirconia copings for all-ceramic crowns: a clinical report. J Prosthet Dent 2008;99(3): 163–73.

81. Lorenzoni FC, Martins LM, Silva NR, et al. Fatigue life and failure modes of crowns systems with a modified framework design. J Dent 2010;38(8):626–34.
82. Rosentritt M, Steiger D, Behr M, et al. Influence of substructure design and spacer settings on the in vitro performance of molar zirconia crowns. J Dent 2009;37(12):978–83.
83. Tinschert J, Schulze KA, Natt G, et al. Clinical behavior of zirconia-based fixed partial dentures made of DC-Zirkon: 3-year results. Int J Prosthodont 2008; 21(3):217–22.
84. Nothdurft FP, Pospiech PR. Zirconium dioxide implant abutments for posterior single-tooth replacement: first results. J Periodontol 2009;80(12):2065–72.
85. Luthardt RG, Holzhuter MS, Rudolph H, et al. CAD/CAM-machining effects on Y-TZP zirconia. Dent Mater 2004;20(7):655–62.
86. Zhang Y, Lawn BR, Rekow ED, et al. Effect of sandblasting on the long-term performance of dental ceramics. J Biomed Mater Res B Appl Biomater 2004; 71(2):381–6.
87. Zhang Y, Lawn BR, Malament KA, et al. Damage accumulation and fatigue life of particle-abraded ceramics. Int J Prosthodont 2006;19(5):442–8.
88. Wang H, Aboushelib MN, Feilzer AJ. Strength influencing variables on CAD/CAM zirconia frameworks. Dent Mater 2008;24(5):633–8.
89. Sato H, Yamada K, Pezzotti G, et al. Mechanical properties of dental zirconia ceramics changed with sandblasting and heat treatment. Dent Mater J 2008; 27(3):408–14.
90. Guazzato M, Quach L, Albakry M, et al. Influence of surface and heat treatments on the flexural strength of Y-TZP dental ceramic. J Dent 2005;33(1):9–18.
91. Kosmac T, Oblak C, Jevnikar P, et al. The effect of surface grinding and sandblasting on flexural strength and reliability of Y-TZP zirconia ceramic. Dent Mater 1999;15(6):426–33.
92. Kosmac T, Oblak C, Jevnikar P, et al. Strength and reliability of surface treated Y-TZP dental ceramics. J Biomed Mater Res 2000;53(4):304–13.
93. Guess PC, Zhang Y, Kim JW, et al. Damage and reliability of Y-TZP after cementation surface treatment. J Dent Res 2010;89(6):592–6.
94. Hickel R, Roulet JF, Bayne S, et al. Recommendations for conducting controlled clinical studies of dental restorative materials. J Adhes Dent 2007;9(Suppl 1): 121–47.
95. Kelly JR. Perspectives on strength. Dent Mater 1995;11(2):103–10.
96. Kelly JR. Clinically relevant approach to failure testing of all-ceramic restorations. J Prosthet Dent 1999;81(6):652–61.
97. Suttor D, Bunke K, Hoescheler S, et al. LAVA–the system for all-ceramic ZrO2 crown and bridge frameworks. Int J Comput Dent 2001;4(3):195–206.
98. Coelho PG, Bonfante EA, Silva NR, et al. Laboratory simulation of Y-TZP all-ceramic crown clinical failures. J Dent Res 2009;88(4):382–6.
99. Guess PC, Zavanelli RA, Silva NR, et al. Monolithic CD/CAM lithium disilicate versus veneered Y-TZP crowns: comparison of failure modes and reliability after fatigue. Int J Prosthodont 2010;23:434–42.
100. Coelho PG, Silva NR, Bonfante EA, et al. Fatigue testing of two porcelain-zirconia all-ceramic crown systems. Dent Mater 2009;25(9):1122–7.
101. Drummond J, Eliades G. Ceramic behavior under different environmental and loading conditions. Dental materials in vivo: aging and related phenomena. Chicago: Quintessence; 2003.
102. Wolf D, Bindl A, Schmidlin PR, et al. Strength of CAD/CAM-generated esthetic ceramic molar implant crowns. Int J Oral Maxillofac Implants 2008;23(4):609–17.

103. Pjetursson BE, Sailer I, Zwahlen M, et al. A systematic review of the survival and complication rates of all-ceramic and metal-ceramic reconstructions after an observation period of at least 3 years. Part I. Single crowns. Clin Oral Implants Res 2007;18(Suppl 3):73–85.

104. Sailer I, Pjetursson BE, Zwahlen M, et al. A systematic review of the survival and complication rates of all-ceramic and metal-ceramic reconstructions after an observation period of at least 3 years. Part II. Fixed dental prostheses. Clin Oral Implants Res 2007;18(Suppl 3):86–96.

105. Napankangas R, Raustia A. Twenty-year follow-up of metal-ceramic single crowns: a retrospective study. Int J Prosthodont 2008;21(4):307–11.

106. Zhang Y, Kim JW. Graded structures for damage resistant and aesthetic all-ceramic restorations. Dent Mater 2009;25(6):781–90.

107. Beuer F, Schweiger J, Eichberger M, et al. High-strength CAD/CAM-fabricated veneering material sintered to zirconia copings–a new fabrication mode for all-ceramic restorations. Dent Mater 2009;25(1):121–8.

108. Groten M, Huttig F. The performance of zirconium dioxide crowns: a clinical follow-up. Int J Prosthodont 2010;23(5):429–31.

109. Schmitt J, Wichmann M, Holst S, et al. Restoring severely compromised anterior teeth with zirconia crowns and feather-edged margin preparations: a 3-year follow-up of a prospective clinical trial. Int J Prosthodont 2010;23(2):107–9.

110. Tsumita M, Kokubo Y, Ohkubo C, et al. Clinical evaluation of posterior all-ceramic FPDs (Cercon): a prospective clinical pilot study. J Prosthodont Res 2010;54(2):102–5.

111. Crisp RJ, Cowan AJ, Lamb J, et al. A clinical evaluation of all-ceramic bridges placed in UK general dental practices: first-year results. Br Dent J 2008;205(9):477–82.

112. Raigrodski AJ, Chiche GJ, Potiket N, et al. The efficacy of posterior three-unit zirconium-oxide-based ceramic fixed partial dental prostheses: a prospective clinical pilot study. J Prosthet Dent 2006;96(4):237–44.

113. Schmitt J, Holst S, Wichmann M, et al. Zirconia posterior fixed partial dentures: a prospective clinical 3-year follow-up. Int J Prosthodont 2009;22(6):597–603.

114. Vult von Steyern P, Carlson P, Nilner K. All-ceramic fixed partial dentures designed according to the DC-Zirkon technique. A 2-year clinical study. J Oral Rehabil 2005;32(3):180–7.

115. Edelhoff D, Florian B, Florian W, et al. HIP zirconia fixed partial dentures–clinical results after 3 years of clinical service. Quintessence Int 2008;39(6):459–71.

116. Molin MK, Karlsson SL. Five-year clinical prospective evaluation of zirconia-based Denzir 3-unit FPDs. Int J Prosthodont 2008;21(3):223–7.

Minimum Thickness Anterior Porcelain Restorations

Gary M. Radz, DDS[a,b,*]

KEYWORDS

- Porcelain laminate veneers • Dental ceramics
- Minimum thickness anterior restorations
- Porcelain restorations

The treatment of healthy but unesthetic teeth has always presented a challenge for the dental practitioner. The introduction of the acid-etch technique by Buonocore[1] and the development of composite resin by Bowen[2] expanded the options for treatment of healthy teeth that were of improper shape, deficient in size, or unesthetic in color. These initial discoveries followed by the work of many others brought to light the possibility of enhancing teeth with porcelain laminate veneers (PLVs).

Since the early 1980s, the development and application of porcelain bonded to tooth restoration using a PLV has enjoyed widespread enthusiasm and success and has now become a widely accepted and popular procedure.

PLVs provide the dentist and the patient with an opportunity to enhance the patient's smile in a minimally to virtually noninvasive manner. Today's PLV demonstrates excellent clinical performance and as materials and techniques have evolved, the PLV has become one of the most predictable, most esthetic, and least invasive modalities of treatment. This article explores the latest porcelain materials and their use in minimum thickness restoration.

HISTORY

The evolution and development of adhesive technology over the past 50 years has provided the foundation for today's veneering techniques. The combination of Buonocore's acid etch research[1] and Bowen's composite resin findings[2] had made possible the technology that allows for the bonding of composite resin to tooth structure in a predictable manner.

In 1928, C.L. Pincus[3] introduced the "Hollywood Veneer." This veneer was not dissimilar from today's porcelain veneers, except that they were not etched, but rather held to place with denture adhesive. Obviously, retention was a significant issue and

[a] Private Practice, 999 18th Street, #1300 Denver, CO 80202, USA
[b] University of Colorado School of Dental Medicine, 10365 East 17th Avenue, Aurora, CO, USA
* Private Practice, 999 18th Street, #1300 Denver, CO 80202.
E-mail address: radzdds@aol.com

Dent Clin N Am 55 (2011) 353–370
doi:10.1016/j.cden.2011.01.006
0011-8532/11/$ – see front matter © 2011 Elsevier Inc. All rights reserved.

these restorations were basically for a temporary cosmetic change for actors to be used in filming and still photography. They needed to be removed before eating and were not functionally sound.

This was then followed by an acrylic resin veneering technique using a chemical bond between the composite resin, now used as cement, and a thin acrylic veneer.[4,5] These veneers were fabricated using indirect acrylic and were bonded to the etched enamel using an ultraviolet light–cured composite resin as the cementing medium.

Introduced in 1979, the Mastique laminate veneer system (caulk) was the first commercially available, mass-produced attempt to bring a veneering system to the market. Preformed acrylic veneers were selected and bonded to the teeth.[6]

In time, the use of an acrylic system for veneering proved to be unsuccessful in the long term. The chemical bond was a weak link leading to debonding and/or fractures. Additionally, esthetically the acrylic lacked the ability to truly simulate tooth structure in either appearance or in function to abrasive forces.[6,7]

Porcelain, however, had a long history as a restorative material in dentistry. Its ability to simulate the optical properties of tooth structure, color stability, stain, and wear resistance along with its history of biocompatibility warranted a search to find a mechanism of attachment to the enamel that would be durable.

Simonsen and Calamia[8–10] provided the initial studies to demonstrate that porcelain etched with hydrofluoric acid could be bonded to composite, which in turn was bonded to etched enamel. Additionally, they demonstrated that this bond would be further enhanced using a silane coupling agent. These studies created the foundation that is still used today in the laboratory fabrication of PLVs and how they are adhesively attached to etched tooth structure. Further studies confirmed these findings.[11,12]

Initially, PLVs were used in a "no-prep" manner.[13] The PLVs were fabricated from stacked feldspathic porcelain. These porcelain veneers were typically 0.5 to 0.7 mm in thickness. The concept was that these restorations were elective/cosmetic in nature and that a noninvasive approach would be ideal. Although the ethical approach of not wanting to remove healthy tooth structure was admirable, it often provided less than desirable results. The veneers often appeared bulky and the soft tissue would show signs of irritation.

As PLVs continued to evolve, a minimally invasive approach was used to provide a more esthetic and biologically compatible restoration. A minimal preparation of 0.5 mm was used to allow for room to place a 0.5- to 0.7-mm-thick piece of porcelain over the tooth. The 0.5 to 0.7 mm of preparation is needed to be able to adequately mask unesthetic areas and/or change the color as well as provide the minimal strength needed for the fabrication and delivery of the PLV.[14,15]

The method of stacking feldspathic porcelain using either a platinum foil technique or refractory die is time intensive and labor intensive and requires a skilled and experienced ceramist. Additionally, stacked porcelain is a fragile material. In an effort to provide a stronger porcelain veneer that was easier for more ceramists to produce, the industry introduced pressed ceramics in 1991 using a leucite-reinforced glass.[16] Using a "lost-wax" technique in combination with staining and/or a cut back and add technique, ceramists now had a system that had more strength, was easier to fabricate, and had excellent esthetic potential. Now more ceramists could meet the esthetic requirements of the practitioner and the patient.

Pressed ceramics (examples: Empress by Ivoclar [Amherst, NY, USA], OPC by Pentron Ceramics [Somerset, NJ, USA]) gained great popularity in the mid 1990s and into the early 2000s, as dentists found great success in providing their patients with highly esthetic results.

This success did not come without some sacrifice. Early leucite-reinforced restorations had to be fabricated in a greater thickness than stacked porcelain. Typical reduction requirements of the time recommended 1.0 mm of reduction.[16] This more aggressive reduction now created a tooth preparation that was mostly in dentin. So the problem created was twofold. First, the ability to bond to dentin is not as predictable or as strong as the bond to enamel.[17–19] Therefore, debondings became more common. Second, the more aggressive removal of tooth structure was found to be very concerning to dentists and patients alike. Concerns were expressed within the dental community questioning the ethics of sacrificing healthy tooth structure for purely esthetic gains.[20–24]

In reaction to this concern by dentists and patients, there was an evolution to return to the initial minimal prep design and there was even a movement to revisit the original no-prep concepts.

Past clinical experience and almost 30 years of data show that PLVs are very predictable and successful when the PLV is bonded to enamel.[25–27] Current best practices in use of PLV for creating an esthetic change is to use a very minimal, if not noninvasive, tooth preparation that is restored with a very thin piece of porcelain. Selecting the proper materials, good case selection, proper techniques, and partnering with a talented ceramist are cornerstones to successful outcomes with PLV therapy.

Indications for PLV

PLV should be used as a conservative solution to an esthetic problem.[28] They are primarily indicated for teeth that are discolored, have displeasing shapes or contours, lack of size and/or volume, or to eliminate diastemata. Additionally, porcelain veneers can have a place in the restoration of loss of tooth structure owing to disease or trauma.

In 2002, Magne and Belser[28] presented the following classification for indications for PLV:

Type I: Teeth resistant to bleaching
  Type IA: Tetracycline discoloration
  Type IB: Teeth that are unresponsive to bleaching

Type II: Major morphologic modifications
  Type IIA: Conoid teeth (peg laterals)
  Type IIB: Diastemata or interdental triangles to be closed
  Type IIC: Augmentation of incisal length or facial prominence (contour)

Type III: Extensive restorations
  Type IIIA: Extensive coronal fracture
  Type IIIB: Extensive loss of enamel by erosion and wear
  Type IIIC: Generalized congenital malformations.

Within Magne and Belser's classification system[28] the use of minimal-preparation and no-preparation porcelain veneers can achieve the desired esthetic outcome in a conservative manner for Types I and II.

Type III cases are more extensive in nature and the treatment goals have as much to do with returning to proper function as they do with esthetics. The use of more aggressive preparation may be necessary to achieve predictable functional results. In many of these cases, the use of stacked ceramics would often not be the first choice. These more extensive restorations would benefit from the stronger leucite-reinforced or lithium disilicate materials now available.

Contraindications

The following are contraindications to use of PLVs:
1. Teeth exposed to heavy occlusal forces, eg, moderate to severe wear owing to bruxism[3]

2. Severely malpositioned teeth
3. Presence of soft tissue disease
4. Highly fluoridated teeth: such teeth may resist acid demineralization and give rise to retention issues
5. Teeth in which color modification can be successfully achieved with various bleaching techniques
6. Teeth with extensive existing restorations.

In cases of minor incisal wear owing to bruxism, it is often possible to restore the incisal length using PLVs. However, it is imperative that the dentist evaluates the occlusal scheme and manages the occlusal forces before any treatment with PLVs is attempted.[29] Many times in these types of cases an occlusal guard is indicated to assist in the prevention of porcelain fracture postoperatively. Excellent patient communication is required before starting such as case.

In cases of misalignment, it is an ethical obligation to discuss the use of orthodontics to create proper alignment. The noninvasive nature of orthodontics will constantly be a better treatment option than any option that includes removal of healthy tooth structure. In the late 1990s, the term "instant orthodontics" was often used to describe PLV therapy as a treatment option for misaligned teeth.[30] This is an aggressive treatment that has been hotly debated in recent years.[31] Although possible to create the illusion of properly aligned teeth with PLVs, it can be a very invasive treatment option that the dentist and the patient need to be very clear on the risks/benefits involved before any treatment is started.

It is important during the treatment-planning and the case-presentation phase of treatment that the dentist provides all the treatment options available and the risks and benefits of these options. PLVs are a versatile restoration that can be a solution to many problems, but they may not always be the best solution. Good judgment and great communication are part of the keys to success with PLV therapy.

Case Selection and Treatment Planning

The key to success with PLVs is in the case selection. The dentist needs to be able to discern those patients who present with conditions that will accept PLVs and have excellent longevity and esthetics; but even more important is learning to identify those cases that are beyond the limits of PLV therapy.

Situations that lend to having good long-term results are patients who have:

1. A well-developed occlusal arch form
2. A balanced and aligned occlusion
3. Postorthodontic treatment
4. Spacing between teeth (diastema)
5. Discolored dentition
6. Symmetric gingival architecture
7. Minimal to no existing anterior restorations.

The absence of any of the listed factors will add to the risk of having a less than desirable esthetic and/or functional result. There are many patients who meet the listed criteria and can benefit from PLV therapy (**Fig. 1**).

Situations that complicate or contraindicate PLVs are:

1. Crowded and/or rotated teeth
2. Narrow occlusal arch form
3. Large existing restorations and/or existing veneers that are bonded to dentin

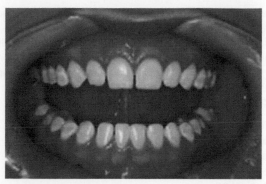

Fig. 1. A postorthodontic 18-year-old patient who is a good candidate for PLV using a minimally invasive approach.

4. Presence of moderate to extreme wear
5. End-to-end anterior occlusion
6. Anterior crossbite
7. Active soft tissue disease
8. Gingival asymmetry
9. History of occlusal or joint dysfunction
10. Psychological issues associated with self-image.

The dentist must carefully evaluate each patient when discussing PLV therapy. There are many patients who would like to have their smiles enhanced using PLV, but not all patients are good candidates for this procedure (**Fig. 2**). For many patients, orthodontics and/or composite bonding, and/or bleaching can be a better treatment option(s).

Proper case selection and excellent communication skills are foundational skills for a dentist to become proficient and successful at providing PLV.

Diagnostics and Records

Once it has been determined that a patient is a good candidate for PLV treatment, it is imperative that a complete oral examination is completed to determine the appropriateness of veneer therapy.

A records appointment is required to provide a complete evaluation of the patient's oral health and to confirm that the patient is indeed a good candidate for this elective

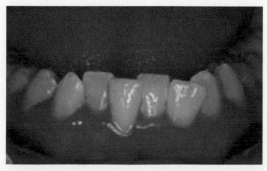

Fig. 2. Crowded and rotated teeth are poor candidates for PLV treatment. Such situations are better served using orthodontic treatment.

treatment. All aspects of the patient's dentition, periodontium, osseous support, joint and muscle health, and extraoral soft tissue need to be evaluated.

A records appointment is required to establish the patient's baseline oral health, to determine the appropriateness of providing the requested restoration(s), and to determine the need for other dental specialty consultations and/or therapies before treatment is started.

The records appointment consists of:

1. Full-mouth radiographs with or without a panoramic radiograph
2. Full-mouth periodontal probing
3. Charting of existing restorations
4. Complete hard and soft tissue evaluation
5. Occlusal/joint evaluation
6. Upper and lower impressions for study model fabrication
7. Bite registration; a facebow transfer may or may not be used for mounting on an articulator
8. Intra- and extraoral photography using American Academy of Cosmetic Dentistry protocol[32]
9. Interview patient regarding goals and expectations.

This information is critical for the dentist to evaluate the appropriateness of the proposed treatment, but it also provides the critical information to develop the treatment plan and the treatment sequence.

Using the information gathered from the examination, it may be necessary to provide the patient with therapies to deal with any disease process present before PLV treatment is started. Additionally, it may be required to seek consultation and possibly treatment by a specialist before the patient's oral condition is ready for the beginning of PLV therapy.

The impressions, bite registration, facebow, and photography are used for the next step in the sequence of PLV treatment. The cast is mounted on an articulator and evaluated for the proposed treatment. This evaluation will determine if the proposed treatment is to go forward.

With the mounted casts on the articulator, the teeth to be veneered are waxed up to ideal contour and occlusion (**Fig. 3**). This wax-up serves as an evaluation of the potential esthetic and functional outcome. This wax-up also allows the dentist to show the patient a preview of the expected final outcome. The wax-up can be an excellent communication tool to ensure that the dentist and ceramist have a good understanding of the patient's esthetic goals, and that the patient's goals can be achieved.

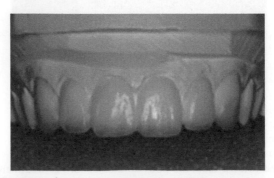

Fig. 3. A diagnostic wax-up for a patient requesting 6 PLVs.

Additionally, this wax-up can be used as a preparation guide and for the fabrication of the patient's temporary veneers.

Preparation

Conventional and current popular practice for conservative PLV preparation is to remove 0.5 mm of tooth structure to create room for the placement of 0.5 mm of porcelain[33–36] on the facial surface. The gingival margin is prepared using a chamfer diamond where the amount of reduction is slightly less, owing to the thinness of the enamel in this area. The gingival margin can be placed supragingival, at the height of tissue, or subgingival. This margin determination is dictated primarily by the esthetic goals. Ideally, subgingival margins should be avoided unless necessary because of the existing tooth color that needs to be blocked out and/or a dramatic change in the higher value of the porcelain shade requested. Last, the incisal edge is prepared by removing 1.0 mm of tooth structure.

Variations and considerations in preparation design

Incisal edge preparation design For many years, experienced clinicians had recommended removing 1.0 mm of tooth structure at the incisal edge, then creating a 1- to 2-mm lingual bevel.[33–36] The idea was that this design would provide stability within the veneer and prevent displacement or cracking of the veneer by functional forces and provide increased overall strength. However, Magne and Belser[28] published convincing evidence that the best incisal preparation design was to remove 1.0 mm of tooth structure at the incisal edge and create a butt-joint margin at the lingual-incisal line angle. Their study concluded that this design best supported the PVL.

Interproximal preparation design No conclusive evidence can be found for what is the best way to prepare the interproximal area of a tooth for a porcelain veneer. Opinions range from virtually no preparation, to a preparation that stops just short of the interproximal contact, to a slight opening of the interproximal contact.

The clinical reality is that each case and each tooth is different. It is up to clinicians to use their best judgment in this area. However, the evidence is clear that margins in enamel are preferred. The margin design here should be such that the margins are not visibly detectable and that a minimum amount of tooth structure should be removed to accomplish this goal.

Preparation guides Over the years, many different ideas have been presented to help the dentist properly and conservatively prepare teeth for PLV. Recently, Magne and Belser[28,37] published a technique to allow for a more conservative approach to PLV preparation.

Frequently the teeth are not in an ideal arch form, and oftentimes to the original facial and/or incisal structure of the tooth has been lost over time.[38] Magne and Belser recommend using a study model to create a wax-up of the ideal final facial, incisal, and lingual contours desired in the final restoration. Then a highly accurate impression of the wax-up is taken using conventional impression material or a silicone putty. This impression now becomes a matrix that will allow the dentist to transfer the wax-up into the patient's mouth using a temporary material (example: LuxaTemp by DMG-America [Englewood, NJ, USA]). This is accomplished by drying the teeth that are to receive PLVs, then loading the matrix with the auto mix temporary material and seating it in the patient's mouth. The temporary material is allowed to set up for 4 to 5 minutes, and then the matrix is removed. The temporary material will adhere to the teeth. With the wax-up (ie, the final desired tooth form/position) now in the patient's mouth, the dentist removes 0.5 mm using a depth-cutting bur to create room for the 0.5-mm-thick PLV. The end result is a more conservative final preparation.

Although it is not always possible to do this procedure in cases of teeth in labial-version or rotated teeth where the rotation carries the tooth facially outside of the ideal arch form, it can provide an excellent general guide for minimizing trauma to the tooth to be prepared.

Ultra-thin preparations In recent years, experienced, skilled ceramists have been able to consistently create PLVs that are 0.3 mm thick. This ability has now allowed many dentists to become even more conservative in their preparation of teeth for PLV. The same previously mentioned preparation guidelines can be used, but now 0.3-mm depth cutters are used to control the preparation depth to an absolute minimum.

Tetracycline and other severe color challenges One of the primary uses of PLVs is to alter the shade of dark-colored teeth. Tetracycline staining and endodontically treated teeth are often esthetic problems for patients.

When treating these patients it is important to have good communication with the patient. Nixon and others[39-44] have demonstrated that it is possible to improve the esthetics on these severely discolored teeth, but the patient needs to be aware of potential compromises. First, it will be very difficult to not have a bit of a graying of the final restoration at the gingival margin. As the porcelain gets thinner at the gingival margin, it becomes increasingly difficult to block out the deeper color of the natural tooth. Second, a slightly more aggressive preparation may be needed to make room for the addition of the opaque porcelains needed to block out this deep color.

Stacked porcelain veneers offer the best solution to get maximum opaquing of the prepared tooth while keeping a minimal preparation. Using stacked porcelain, a thin layer of opacious dentin porcelain can be first laid down to opaque the dark tooth color; then the ceramist can layer the porcelain in such a way as to be able to create the desired results. Pressed ceramics do not offer the same flexibility in technique and would require a slightly more aggressive preparation to achieve similar results.

Impressions and Bite Registration

Once the preparations have been completed, the final impression can be obtained. Currently polyethers and vinylpolysiloxanes (VPS) are the most popular materials for final impressions. Either type of material can accurately record the intraoral condition.

Retraction cord may or may not be required. Experienced clinicians will often use a very small diameter retraction cord to create a small amount of apical displacement to record the unprepared tooth structure below the prepared margin. The gingival tissues around anterior teeth are often thin and fragile. It is critical to minimize the trauma to this tissue during cord placement.

Recently there has been the introduction of "pastelike" materials (Expisyl by Kerr [Orange, CA, USA]) that can be used to provide slight retraction of the gingival tissue.[45] The atraumatic nature of these materials makes them appealing for this application.

An accurate bite registration is required to be able to accurately mount the working models. There are many different materials on the market today that can accomplish this task.

The horizontal orientation of the maxillary arch is critical information for the ceramist. In cases where the veneers are minimal in their design and the functional occlusion will not be altered as "stick-bite" can be adequate. A "stick-bite" is obtained by having the patient stand up; placing a small amount of VPS bite registration (example: BluMouse by Parkell [Edgewood, NY, USA]) on the incisal surfaces of the anterior teeth, have the patient close, then place a "stick" (often a long cotton tip applicator) into the bite regis-tration. Then the stick is manipulated to being parallel to the horizon.

A more accurate and desirable method is to use a facebow transfer to accurately record the horizontal maxillary position.

It is timely to mention the existence of digital impression technology in many of today's dental offices. Digital impressions can be used for PLV, but if they are used it needs to be in conjunction with a minimum of a "stick-bite" and/or a facebow transfer.

Shade Selection

In cases where PLVs are being placed electively for cosmetic purposes, it is important to get the patient's input. Using shade guides and photographs of previous cases, the dentist can begin to gain an understanding of what the patient is looking to achieve in the final results. It is imperative for the success of these cases that the dentist takes into consideration the patient's goals.

In cases where the PLVs are being used to on 1 to 4 (or even 6) teeth, the dentist now needs to strive to reproduce a restoration(s) that matches the shade of the remaining natural teeth. With a case that will include 8 to 10 teeth in the arch, the shade selection should be an agreement between the dentist and the patient as to what shade will met the patient's goals.

Digital photography can be a helpful tool when communicating with the ceramist. Photographs taken of the prepared teeth at various angles with and without a shade guide in the picture will help the ceramist have a better opportunity to achieve the desired final result.

Another tool commercially available are digital shade taking devices (example: EasyShade by Vident [Brea, CA, USA]). These devices can be used to record the shade of the existing dentition. Caution must be used when using these devices. Although a helpful tool in selecting a shade, they should only be used as an adjunctive method of making the final selection.

Laboratory Communication

For the ceramist to provide the desired final results, it is critical to send him or her as much information as possible to help in the fabrication of the PLV.

The following information should be sent to the laboratory:

1. Final impression (full arch)
2. Impression of the opposing arch (full arch)
3. Bite registration with a stick-bite or facebow transfer
4. Photographs of the preoperative condition and the prepared teeth, as well as shade tabs next to the prepared and unprepared teeth. The photos can be stored on a disc or flash drive or sent via e-mail.
5. Return of the wax-up with a notation if anything has been altered on the wax-up
6. Written laboratory prescription with details on the desired final results and the desired type of porcelain to be used.

Additional information that may sometimes be helpful includes:

1. A study model of the temporary restorations
2. Photographs from magazines or the dentist's own patient library showing smile designs that the dentist and/or the patient may want to try to simulate
3. Diagrams written on a photo or from a "smile design" book.

Material Options

For use as a material for thin, conservative PLVs there are currently 2 options available.

Traditional feldspathic stacked veneers

Feldspathic ceramic is a ceramic that is designed to mimic natural dentition. These porcelains are mainly composed of feldspar, quartz, and kaolin. The blending amounts have been adjusted over years to produce the translucent levels and opaque levels in glass. There are many different types and recipes including use of synthetics. Overall, their properties are similar. Most importantly, when using feldspathic type of porcelain for thin veneers the common denominator is the supporting matrix during fabrication as well as cementation. The refractory die investment and the platinum foil support the porcelain during ceramic firing and grinding because of the overall brittleness and reduced strength, 50 to 90 MPa, in feldspathic porcelain. Once bonded to enamel the material is strengthened by the underlying tooth just as when manufactured on its matrix.

The fabrication of feldspathic veneers requires 1 of 2 different techniques; either the refractory system or the foil system.

The *refractory system* is a technique where a master model is fabricated by pinning the prepared teeth into removable dies. It is then duplicated using a polyvinylsiloxane-duplicating material in a refectory high-heat investment including ceramic die pins. This allows the dies to be fired repeatedly in a porcelain furnace. These dies are first degassed to remove any ammonia in the refectory investment and the feldspathic porcelain is applied to the dies. They are then placed into a ceramic furnace and fired according to the manufacturer's specifications. After the veneers are built and fired, they are contoured and form and function are refined. The veneers are then glazed and polished. The refectory investment material is removed from the veneers by air abrading with 50 μm of aluminous oxide. The veneers are then transferred to the master dies for reexamination of fit and function.

The *foil technique* is the fabrication of veneers using a 0.001 dead soft platinum foil that is adapted to the master dies.[46] The platinum foil is burnished by hand with a tool and swedged in a clay-filled cylinder to achieve premium adaptation. The feldspathic porcelain is applied directly to the foil substrate and placed in the ceramic furnace for firing. The veneers are then contoured and refined on the master model to optimum form and function. The veneers are then glazed and polished. The platinum foil is then teased out of the inside of the veneers and transferred to the master model for final refinements.

Pressed lithium disilicate

Lithium disilicate is composed of quartz, lithium dioxide, phosphor oxide, alumina, potassium oxide, and other components. These materials are combined in a glass melt. Once proper viscosity is achieved, it is placed in steel molds and cooled. Overall, this composition yields a highly thermal shock-resistant glass ceramic owing to low thermal expansion when it is manufactured. This allows for self-supporting strength during fabrication. Lithium disilicate is rated at approximately 400 MPa.

Pressed thin veneers using lithium disilicate are fabricated using a lost-wax technique. The master model is fabricated with the preparations cut into dies. The tissue is trimmed from the model, the dies are sealed, and a layer of spacer is added. The veneers are waxed to full contour. They are then sprued and invested in a ring of pressing high-heat investment. The rings are placed in a burnout oven where the wax melts out leaving a mold of the restorations. The mold then has an ingot placed inside and a plunger is placed into a porcelain press where the molten glass is pressed into the mold under vacuum pressure. The molds are divested using glass beads in an air abrasion unit. The lithium disilicate veneers are cut off of the sprue leads and placed in a 1% hydrofluoric acid solution for 10 to 15 minutes to remove the reaction layer. The pressings are then fit to the master dies, and sprues are ground off and contoured. The veneers are either custom stained or micro-layered with a fluorapatite-based layering ceramic.[47] The veneers are evaluated for form and function on the master cast. Last, they are refined and glazed and polished.

Temporization

Throughout the years, one of the biggest challenges presented with a porcelain veneer case was the question of how to successfully provide a provisional restoration. Many different techniques and materials have been used with various levels of success.

Currently one of the most popular and predictable techniques is to start with a wax-up of the desired final results. This wax-up will be used for the Magne/Belser preparation guide. The silicone putty or VPS putty matrix created from the wax-up is also used as the matrix for the temporary restorations.

Once the final impression(s) and bite registration have been taken, the patient is now ready for temporization. The prepared teeth are isolated and dried. The preparations are then spot-etched using phosphoric acid in the middle of each prepared tooth. The etchant is allowed to stay on the teeth for 30 seconds, then teeth are rinsed and dried. A small amount of a lightly filled resin (example: the second bottle of the Optibond FL bonding agent by Kerr) is placed on the area of the preparation(s) that was etched. The bonding agent is then light cured for 5 to 10 seconds.

Next the putty matrix is loaded with an auto mix temporary material (example: Lux-atemp by DMG-America) using a shade that is in the approximate range of the final restorations. This matrix is then inserted into the mouth and allowed to sit for at least 5 minutes.

When the matrix is removed, a highly detailed, esthetic duplication of the wax-up is now in place as the patient's provisional restoration. Not only does this provide patients with a socially acceptable, esthetic smile, it also gives them a preview of the final restorations.

It will be necessary to trim off the excess temporary material. At the gingival margins a 16-fluted carbide bur and a #12 scalpel blade can be used to carefully, atraumatically remove excess temporary material. The #12 blade is an excellent tool for removing material in the interproximal areas. A 16-fluted "football"-shaped carbide is used to remove any excess material on the lingual, and is also used to adjust and refine the occlusion.

Finishing of the temporary material can be accomplished with any number of composite finishing instruments.

A highly esthetic final polish can be obtained using a prophy cup and composite polishing paste.

When doing multiple units, it is advisable and acceptable to leave the restoration in one unit that will splint all the prepared teeth. By using this splinting process, the provisional veneers have improved retention. However, it is critical when this technique is used that great care is taken to finishing the papilla area and allow from room to use a floss threader for home care (**Fig. 4**).

Try-in

When the veneer return to the office from the laboratory, the dentist should take the time to evaluate the case to be sure that his or her directions have been followed and expectations have been met.

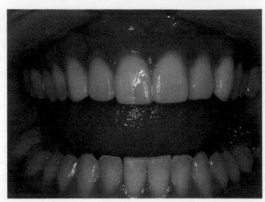

Fig. 4. Direct bonded provisional veneers can provide excellent esthetics and soft tissue health. Provisional veneers are on #'s 6–11 and have been in place for 6 weeks.

When the patient returns to the office, the temporary restorations are removed. The preparations are cleaned with a prophy cup and a slurry of pumice.

Ideally, the color of the veneers will be built into the porcelain as well as, frequently, from the color of the natural tooth underneath. For this reason, the veneers should first be tried in using a translucent try-in paste. Try-in pastes are water-soluble pastes that are designed to simulate the color that is present in the final cements. The try-in pastes also act as a weak adhesive to allow the dentist and patient an opportunity to evaluate the PLV.

It is critical at this point to get the patient's feedback. As oftentimes this is an elective procedure, the patient's input at this point is important. It is much easier to send the veneers back at the try-in phase as opposed to having bonded them to place and only then find out the patient does not like the esthetics.

At this time, it is possible to make subtle shifts in the shade of the veneer by using colored cements. The try in pastes allow for the dentist to evaluate shade modifications. Oftentimes the use of a colored cement will allow the dentist to create the desired color.

Once the dentist has evaluated fit, and together with the patient evaluated the shade and contours, a determination is made as to whether or not the veneers will be delivered at this appointment.

Cementation

The teeth to receive the PLV restorations are first isolated with a rubber dam. The preparations are cleaned again with a slurry of pumice and a prophy cup.

Fluid control is critical at this point. Any hemorrhage present must be under control. Various methods are available to do this: aluminum chloride solutions, retraction pastes that contain aluminum chloride, retraction cord with epinephrine, direct infiltration of local anesthetic that contains epinephrine, and/or a diode laser.

Much discussion has occurred since PLVs have existed as to how many veneers to place at one time. Even today there are those who firmly believe that veneers should be placed 2 at a time starting with the centrals; then there are other clinicians who advocate placing all of the veneers at the same time. Each of these techniques has challenges. Dentists must base this decision on their own experience/comfort level, the difficulty of the case, and the total number of PLVs to be placed.

With the teeth isolated, a 35% to 37% phosphoric etch solution is placed on the prepared teeth. The etchant is left on the teeth for a minimum of 30 seconds. The etchant is then rinsed and dried. It should be noted at this time that it is assumed that a vast majority of the prepared tooth surface is enamel. With this assumption, it is acceptable to etch for longer periods of time, and concerns about desiccation of the tooth do not apply to an all-enamel preparation.

Next, a total-etch bonding agent, either fourth or fifth generation (examples: Optibond FL by Kerr, Prime & Bond NT by Caulk [Milford, DE, USA]), is applied to the preparation(s) as per the manufacturer's directions.

The bonding solution is then air thinned and light cured for a minimum of 10 seconds per tooth using an appropriate light source.

The veneers are then individually loaded with the light-cure resin cement of choice (example: Variolink by Ivoclar) using the shade selected at try-in. Because of the thinness of these veneers, there should be no need to use dual-cure resin cement. By using a light-cure only material, any concerns about shade shift associated with dual-cure resins becomes irrelevant.

The veneers are carefully seated to place, excess cement is removed, and each veneer is light cured for a total of 60 seconds.

Finishing and Polishing

Upon completion of the cementation there will be some excess resin cement that will need to be removed.

Initial removal from the gingival and the interproximal can be achieved with a #12 scalpel blade. Additionally, a 12- or 16-fluted carbide can be used in these areas, and a "football"-shaped carbide is ideally shaped to remove excess on the lingual.

With thin PLV, there are occasions when the porcelain will be bulky on the margins. In these areas, a fine diamond with a light water spray can be used to carefully reshape the porcelain.

Interproximally, fine diamond strips followed by a series of aluminum oxide finishing strips can be used to remove excess resin cement and then polish.

The facial and lingual margins that have been adjusted can now be repolished. Haywood and colleagues[48] showed that porcelain adjustments made with a fine diamond and water spray, followed by 30-fluted carbide without water at high RPMs, and polished with a series of porcelain polishing points/discs can return a surface texture that rivals glazed porcelain. This polishing technique should also be used on any lingual areas that have been adjusted for occlusal reasons.

Postoperative Appointment

For any large case, a postoperative appointment is necessary. In the case of a patient with PLVs, the postoperative appointment has several purposes:

1. Evaluate the occlusion and make any necessary adjustments.
2. Evaluate the soft tissue health.
   a. Interproximally the veneer margins are checked using dental floss. Any place where the floss shreds indicates that excess cement is present. This can be removed and polished using aluminum oxide finishing strips.
   b. Gingivally, the soft tissue at the margins is evaluated for any signs of irritation. Irritation can indicate the presence of excess cement, which can be removed with a #12 scalpel blade or a 16-fluted carbide bur. The irritation could also indicate an area that is overcontoured. An overcontoured area can be adjusted using a fine diamond, then repolishing the area.

3. Postoperative photographs should be taken at this time for documentation of the case.
4. If an occlusal splint is indicated for the patient, it is at this appointment when the impressions are taken.
5. Last, the patient is given home-care instructions to help maximize the life span of the restorations.

THE NO-PREP OPTION

During the infancy of PLVs, a no-prep approach was used by dentists. This approach fell into disuse as the esthetic results were not optimal and dentist and ceramist found they could create a better final result by using a minimal preparation design.

In the past decade, partially driven by dentists concerned about the amount of healthy tooth structure that was being sacrificed for purely cosmetic reasons and partially driven by patients' desires to improve their appearance without having parts of their teeth removed, there has been a resurgence of the no-prep design.

Marketing efforts directed to the consumer created a great demand by the patient population. However, many dentists were concerned with the final results being bulky, opaque, and the potential for soft tissue irritation. Dentists were also concerned about the potential for abuse of this treatment option (**Fig. 5**A). Debate still continues on the viability of no-prep veneers.[49] Although most all dentists agree that it is desirable to cosmetically restore teeth without removing healthy tooth structure, the debate continues as to whether or not it is possible to achieve the desired esthetics and have long-term function and soft tissue health.

Recently Wells[50] and others have demonstrated that in certain situations it is possible to place no-prep veneers while achieving the desired esthetic results without compromising function of soft tissue health.

Case Selection

Case selection is critical for the success of a no-prep veneer. Wells provides the following guidelines[51]:

1. Microdontia, such as peg laterals, tooth width and arch form discrepancies, and in general, undersized teeth.
2. Short, worn teeth that have lost some volume owing to occlusal wear, abrasion, erosion, or some combination of these factors.
3. Bicuspid extraction orthodontic cases where anterior teeth are lingui-verted and the arch form is narrow.
4. Large lips that create a big "frame" and allow enlargement (addition of volume) of the teeth for proper proportion.

Fig. 5B demonstrates a patient with very full lips. The fullness of the lips allows for the potential to add facial volume to the teeth without compromising the final esthetic result.

The final determination as to whether or not a patient is a good candidate for a no-prep PVL is to place a prototype of the final desired result on the tooth. Wells[51] discussed the use of a direct-bonded composite prototype. Spot etching the teeth with phosphoric acid on each tooth that is being considered for a no-prep PLV is recreated using composite resin. The composite resin is fabricated directly onto the tooth and finished and polished to simulate the desired final result. This prototype allows the dentist and the patient to evaluate the final result before the PLVs are ever fabricated. If the direct-bonded prototypes are found acceptable by the patient

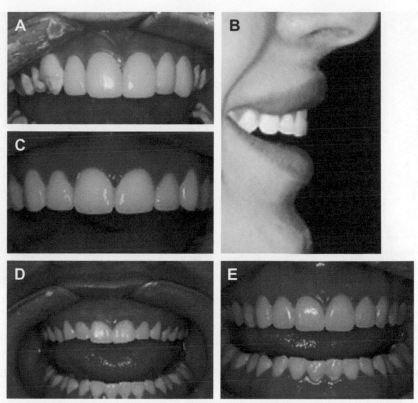

Fig. 5. (*A*) No-prep veneers placed 8 weeks previously on 8 teeth on a 14-year-old patient. (*B*) Patient profile demonstrating full lips that can tolerate the addition of volume provided by no-prep veneers. (*C*) No-prep veneers on the canines and laterals at a 2-year postoperative visit. (*D*) Preoperative view of patient to receive 10 maxillary lithium disilicate (eMax, Ivoclar) no-prep PLVs. (*E*) Patient with 10 maxillary lithium disilicate (eMax, Ivoclar) noprep PLVs at 2 months postoperative.

and the dentist, an impression is made of the prototypes and sent to the ceramist for duplication in porcelain.

A similar, yet less accurate method would be to create a wax-up, then using Magne and Belser's technique[28] described earlier for use as a preparation guide, transfer the wax up into the patients mouth using an automix temporary material (example: Luxa-Temp by DMG-America). The temporary material can be finished and polished to provide a similar preview of the desired final result.

Once it has been determined that the patient is a good candidate for no-prep veneers using a prototyping technique, the steps to completion remain the same. The previously listed information is required by the ceramist; try-in and delivery techniques remain the same. The only difference is after cementation there will always be a need to refine the gingival margins of a no-prep veneer. The physical limitations of porcelain will leave a small bit of excess porcelain at the margin. Wells[51] describes a finishing and polishing technique using fine diamonds with a water spay and magnification to minimize the bulk at the gingival margin. This is followed by polishing with a 30-fluted carbide[48] and completed using a series of rubber polishers and diamond polishing paste on a Robinson bristle brush. Using this technique, it is possible to finish

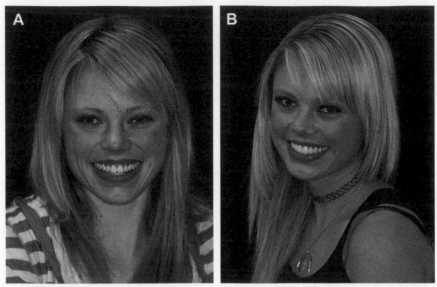

Fig. 6. (*A, Before*) A young patient with discolored and unesthetic smile. (*B, After*) The patients smile is restored in a conservative manner using minimal and no preparation pressed ceramic (eMax, Ivoclar) veneers.

the PLV margins to a contour and smoothness that will allow for excellent esthetics and desired soft tissue health.

Fig. 5C is a 2-year postoperative photograph of no-prep porcelain veneers on the canines and laterals demonstrating the esthetic and soft tissue results that can be obtained.

Originally no-prep veneers were created strictly using stacked porcelain; however, it has been shown that lithium disilicate (eMax, Ivoclar) can also be used to create excellent results now that this material has the ability to be used in very thin layers (see **Fig. 5**D, E).[52]

When the proper criteria are followed, along with excellent ceramic work and good clinical technique, it is possible to provide excellent results with no-prep porcelain veneers.

SUMMARY

PLVs when done using proper materials and techniques and used in a conservative manner have proven to be a highly successful form of treatment. PLV therapy should not be misunderstood as a treatment only for the vain. A person's self-esteem can be directly related to the appearance of his or her smile. Additionally, how others respond to a person with a pleasing smile versus a person with an unesthetic smile can be vastly different.

With PLVs we are not only helping people improve the appearance of their smile, we are also providing psychological and social benefits. The importance of this is difficult to measure. But ask people who have benefited from having PLVs used to enhance their smiles and I'm sure they will tell you of the significant impact it has had for them (**Fig. 6**).

ACKNOWLEDGMENTS

The ceramic work presented in this article was created by Americus Dental Labs (NY), Dental Arts Lab (IL), and YES Dental Lab (NY).

REFERENCES

1. Buonocore MG. A simple method of increasing the adhesion of acrylic filling materials to enamel surfaces. J Dent Res 1955;34:849–53.
2. Bowen RL. Development of a silica-resin direct filling material. Report 6333. Washington, DC: National Bureau of Standards; 1958.
3. Pincus CL. Building mouth personality. J Calif Dent Assoc 1938;14(4):125–9.
4. Faunce RF, Faunce AR. The use of laminate veneers for restoration of fractured discolored teeth. Tex Dent J 1975;98(8):6–7.
5. Faunce RF. Tooth restoration with preformed laminated veneers. J Tex Dent Assoc 1977;53:30.
6. Boyer DB, Chalkley Y. Bonding between acrylic laminates and composite resin. J Dent Res 1982;61:489–92.
7. Cannon ML. In vivo and in vitro abrasion of preformed resin veneers. J Dent Res 1980 [abstract #1093].
8. Simonsen RJ, Calamia JR. Tensile bond strength of etched porcelain. J Dent Res 1983 [abstract #1154].
9. Calamia JR, Simonsen RJ. Effect of coupling agents in bond strength of etched porcelain. J Dent Res 1984;63:179.
10. Calamia JR. Etched porcelain facial veneers: a new treatment modality based on scientific and clinical evidence. N Y J Dent 1983;53(6):255–9.
11. Hsu C, Stangel I, Nathanson D. Shear bond strengths of resin to etched porcelain. J Dent Res 1985 [abstract #1095].
12. Horn HR. Porcelain laminate veneers bonded to etched enamel. Dent Clin North Am 1983;27:671–84.
13. Calamia JR. Etched porcelain veneers: the current state of the art. Quintessence Int 1985;16(1):5–12.
14. Quinn F, McConnell RJ. Porcelain laminates: a review. Br Dent J 1986;161(2):61–5.
15. McClean JW. Ceramics in clinical dentistry. Br Dent J 1988;164:187–94.
16. Nash RW. What's different about IPS empress esthetic. CERP 2005;52–7.
17. Meiers JC, Young D. Two-year composite/dentin durability. Am J Dent 2001;14:141–4.
18. Hashimoto M, Ohno H, Kaga M, et al. Resin-tooth interfaces after long-term function. Am J Dent 2001;14:211–5.
19. Dumfahrt H, Schaffer H. Porcelain laminate veneers: a retrospective evaluation after 1–10 years of service. Int J Prosthodont 2000;13:9–18.
20. Heymann HO. Right on Ron. J Esthet Restor Dent 2007;19(1):1–2.
21. Christensen GJ. Veneer mania. J Am Dent Assoc 2006;137(8):1161–3.
22. Heymann HO, Swift EJ. Is tooth structure not sacred anymore? J Esthet Restor Dent 2001;13(5):1–2.
23. Bakeman EM, Goldstein RE, Sesemann MR. Responsible esthetics: is there a return to conservative esthetic dentistry? Inside Dent 2010;6(6):36.
24. DiMatteo AM. Dissecting the debate over the ethics of esthetic dentistry. Inside Dentistry 2007;3(8):56–8.
25. Friedman MJ. A 15 year review of porcelain veneer failure—a clinician's observation. Compend Contin Educ Dent 1998;19(6):625–38.
26. Strassler HE, Nathanson D. Clinical evaluation of etched porcelain veneers over a period of 18 to 42 months. J Esthet Dent 1989;1(1):21–8.

27. Calamia JR, Calamia CS. Porcelain laminate veneers: reasons for 25 years of success. Dent Clin North Am 2007;51:399–417.
28. Magne P, Belser UC. Bonded porcelain restorations in the anterior dentition—a biomimetic approach. Chicago: Quintessence Publishing Co; 2002.
29. Kois JC. Functional occlusion I: science driven management. Kois Center, Seattle (WA), 2007.
30. Lowe RA. Instant orthodontics: an alternative esthetic option. Dent Prod Rep 2002;36(4):50–2.
31. Jacobson N, Frank CA. The myth of instant orthodontics: an ethical quandary. J Am Dent Assoc 2008;139(4):424–33.
32. American Academy of Cosmetic Dentistry (AACD). A guide to Accreditation photography-photographic documentation and evaluation in cosmetic dentistry. Madison (WI): AACD; 2009.
33. Nash RW. Conservative elective porcelain veneers. Compend Contin Educ Dent 1999;20(9):888–96.
34. Nash RW. Stacked porcelain veneers: a preparation technique. Dent Prod Rep 2002;36(9):54–5.
35. Lerner JM. Conservative aesthetic enhancement of the maxillary anterior region using porcelain laminate veneers. Pract Proced Aesthet Dent 2006;18(6):361–6.
36. Rosenthal L, Rinaldi P. Producing preparation designs in patients who require simultaneous, different restorative protocols. Estht Tech 2001;1(3):1–9.
37. Magne P, Belser UC. Novel porcelain laminate preparation approach driven by a diagnostic mock-up. J Esthet Restor Dent 2004;16:7–18.
38. Magne P, Douglas W. Additive contour of porcelain veneers: a key element in enamel preservation, adhesion, and esthetics for aging dentition. J Adhes Dent 1999;1:81–92.
39. Feinman RA, Nixon RL. Achieving optimal aesthetic for severely stained dentition with laminate veneers. Clinical Contours 1998;2(1):1–7.
40. Okuda WH. Using a modified subopaquing technique to treat highly discolored dentition. J Am Dent Assoc 2000;131:945–50.
41. Nixon RL. Masking severely tetracycline-stained teeth with porcelain veneers. Pract Periodontics Aesthet Dent 1990;2(1):14–8.
42. Dickerson W. Veneer preparation and cementation in tetracycline-stained teeth treatment. CERP 2000;50–4.
43. Nash RW. Tetracycline stain: an esthetic challenge. Dent Prod Rep 2006;56–7.
44. Bassett J, Patrick B. Restoring tetracycline-stained teeth with a conservative preparation for porcelain veneers: case presentation. Pract Proced Aesthet Dent 2004;16(7):481–6.
45. Radz GM. Concepts in soft-tissue management in contemporary dentistry. Available at: www.kerr.dentalaegis.com. Accessed September 5, 2010.
46. Weyandt F, Kahng LS. The benefits of platinum-foil veneering. Cont Estht 2006;26–30.
47. Schwartz JC. Layering technique for pressed ceramic laminate veneers. Pract Proced Aesthet Dent 2002;14(5):381–5.
48. Haywood VB, Heymann HO, Scurria MS. Effects of water, speed and experimental instrumentation on finishing and polishing porcelain intra-orally. Dent Mater 1989;5:185–8.
49. DiMatteo AM. Prep vs no prep: the evolution of veneers. Inside Dentistry 2009;5(6):72–9.
50. Wells DJ. Don't we all do cosmetic dentistry? Dent Econ 2007;97(4):106–9.
51. Wells DJ. "No-prep" veneers. Inside Dent 2010;6(8):56–60.
52. Radz GM. Enhancing the esthetics through addition: no prep porcelain veneers. Oral Health 2009;99(4):23–30.

Creating Aesthetic Success Through Proper Clinician and Laboratory Technical Communication

John F. Weston, DDS[a], Erik Haupt, BA[b],*

KEYWORDS

• Lab communication • Aesthetics • Porcelain • Ceramist

High-quality aesthetic restorations that look great, function ideally, and last can only be predictably produced through implementation of excellent communication techniques and systems between the doctor and ceramist. Often, communication to the laboratory is only thought about at the end of an appointment when the laboratory prescription is being filled out. With the availability of technology and the Internet, it is now easy to involve the laboratory via digital photographs. This article challenges one to begin including the laboratory early in the process and routinely use reliable techniques to transfer clinically significant information to the laboratory bench. It is easy to complete a great case once in a while, but only through developing a system and working together with a quality-conscious ceramist, can a dentist achieve real aesthetic success with every case. Setting the goals with the patient is important and can be a valuable source to review throughout case construction. Including the laboratory in these goals is an essential part of the equation, and reviewing these goals with the patient after completion of the case can be valuable in determining the success or failure of a particular case.

PHOTOGRAPHY

The first and most logical step is to document cases properly through quality photographic views. A single-lens reflex digital camera with a basic ring flash and 50 to 100 mm lens should be used. Having the proper camera system is necessary to create consistent results. The American Academy of Cosmetic Dentistry (AACD) has developed a photography guideline that is helpful in viewing and examining the aesthetic

[a] Scripps Center for Dental Care, 9850 Genesee Avenue, Suite 620, La Jolla, CA 92037, USA
[b] Haupt Dental Laboratory, 1220 East Birch Street # 201, Brea, CA 92821-5155, USA
* Corresponding author.
E-mail address: erik@sbcglobal.net

Dent Clin N Am 55 (2011) 371–382
doi:10.1016/j.cden.2011.01.007
0011-8532/11/$ – see front matter © 2011 Published by Elsevier Inc.

properties of a case. The 12 AACD-required photographs are an excellent starting point toward successful communication (**Figs. 1–3**). Properly exposed and framed photographs allow the ceramist to see what materials and techniques are necessary to create the final result. Additional photographs to consider beyond these would be shade reference views and lips in repose or at rest. Theseare valuable views to determine the final length of the central incisors, which is typically 2 to 3 mm should be displayed beyond the edge of the upper lip (**Fig. 4**). Lastly, it is important that all the photographs are taken with the teeth well hydrated. A tooth that is dehydrated will have a higher value and chroma than a hydrated one. These photographs set the foundation for all successful dentist/ceramist teams.

MODELS

It is always valuable to record the detail of shapes and positions of the natural teeth before providing any treatment via models. Because of the availability of inexpensive polyvinyl siloxane materials, alginate impressions are no longer the standard of care for opposing or preoperative models. The laboratory technician will often refer back to the original teeth many times while building a case to see what features of the patients' teeth need to be incorporated in the new design. Providing accurate and reproducible models is an important issue. Subtle details in texture, anatomy, and contours keep the ceramic restorations from looking contrived and can provide the element of "perfect imperfection" that natural teeth exhibit. One should never underestimate the value of what was working in a patients smile before the case was started. The most beautiful smiles are created in the laboratory by looking for ways to improve what nature provided instead of erasing and rebuilding from scratch.

JAW RELATION RECORDS

There are many theories on the best way to manage restorations with regard to occlusion. There is also a great debate about which theory is right. However, there is no debate about the fact that there should be a consistent method that provides a reliable and repeatable record to mount models and build a case. In the end, the teeth must be able to occlude with function and comfort for sustained periods and not overload the muscles and joints. Having accurate bite records helps to confidently cross-mount all models from preoperative to prepared to provisional, allowing the laboratory technician maximum ability to build an accurate occlusal scheme. Typically, once the reconstruction proceeds beyond the canines, a face bow transfer is indicated. This process

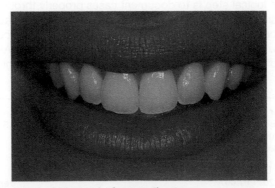

Fig. 1. An AACD-required photograph, front smile view.

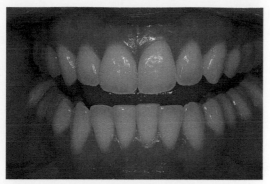

Fig. 2. An AACD-required photograph, front retracted view.

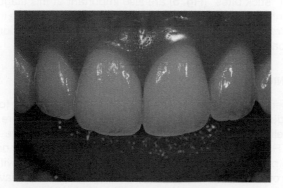

Fig. 3. An AACD required photograph, front close-up view.

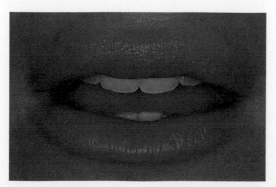

Fig. 4. Properly framed, lips at rest or repose, note proper incisal display.

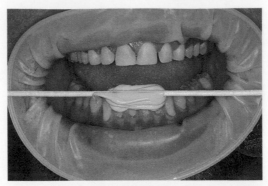

Fig. 5. Stick bite secured to lower teeth, horizontal to the plane of the earth.

requires the laboratory technician and doctor to have the same articulators. The face bow can be transferred to the laboratory by sending the face bow hardware and bite fork mount, or the clinician can simply mount the upper model. Horizontal references, commonly called "stick bites" (**Fig. 5**) are also important at this stage to prevent the formation of a canted midline. Studies show that canted midlines are the most noticed of all midline discrepancies, and mounting the casts properly in relation to the plane of the earth and a patient's face can help prevent this problem.

SHADE COMMUNICATION

Proper shade reference photographs are one of the most important tools for communicating with a dental laboratory. Many dentist/ceramist teams are geographically separated thus eliminating the opportunity for the patient to drive back and forth between offices. Having the final shade incorrect is often the number one issue leading to an unsatisfied patient. Multiple views should be taken with and without retractors, using a selection of shade tabs on hydrated teeth. These views will have the shade tab on a parallel plane with the referenced tooth (**Fig. 6**). It is also important to have the same amount of light on both the shade tab and the referenced tooth. Another important photograph for the laboratory is that of the prepared tooth. Many all-ceramic restorative materials, once seated, are influenced by the preparation shade. The laboratory technician needs to see a photograph of the dentin to appropriately build the intended shade. Using software, the laboratory technician can then digitally

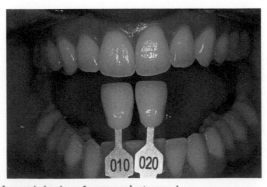

Fig. 6. A properly framed shade reference photograph.

manipulate the images to discern levels of value and chroma (**Fig. 7**). It is also important to make sure that the laboratory technician's and clinician's computer monitors are calibrated so that each person sees the same color combinations. The camera has to be set with proper white balance, f-stop, and flash sync for properly exposed images. As a backup, a color calibration card can be used to make sure that the shade is properly represented in the images that are sent to the laboratory. What may seem intimidating to a dentist is simplified by working with companies that can set up the dental clinical camera, (PhotoMed International, Los Angeles, CA, USA) for consistent results.

DIGITAL SHADE COMMUNICATION

There are also computerized devices that can make shade matching available to even the most color-challenged individuals. A person can literally point the device on the surface of a tooth, and within seconds, a shade will be given on a liquid crystal display screen (**Fig. 8**). Although the shade may not be accurate in every case, it gives a starting point and with the assistance of photography, allows additional ability to extrapolate all the nuances within a tooth.

PORCELAIN CHARACTERIZATION

An important skill required in creating porcelain restorations that appear natural is controlling the amount of characterization. Natural teeth have varying amounts of incisal translucency, and the ceramist needs to recreate this characteristic accurately. What may seem simple often involves more that just placing porcelain across the incisal edge. There are many colors and effects seen within natural teeth that correspond to different incisal porcelain powders. By using examples of teeth from published books the dentist can describe how much, value, chroma, and incisal character they desire. Whether natural teeth or restorations, color photographs of desired characteristics can prove invaluable. Additional information for incisal characterization can be obtained by taking a photograph at a 30° downward angle to the facial plane of the natural tooth (**Fig. 9**). This technique provides an excellent record of incisal translucency.[1]

PREPARATION DESIGN AND MATERIAL SELECTION

The teeth should always be prepared in a way that preserves as much tooth structure as possible. Once the goals of the case are determined, preparations should be

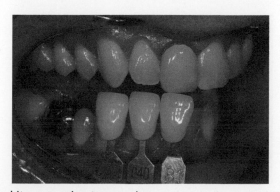

Fig. 7. Black and white conversion to see value.

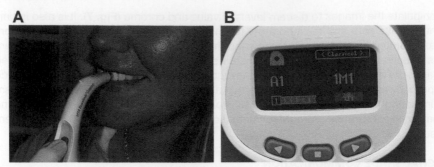

Fig. 8. Easyshade device (VITA Zahnfabrik H. Rauter GmbH & Co. KG, Bad Säckingen, Germany) in use, results are instant (*A, B*).

decided clinically based on design parameters, shade requirements, and available tooth structure. Restorative material choices should be finalized in the laboratory to match the strength and aesthetic goals required by the case while meeting the preparation clearances provided. Blindly preparing teeth just to fit the parameters of certain restoratives could be considered inappropriate and, in some cases, malpractice. Porcelain veneering was initially introduced as a "no prep" procedure. Whereas bonding strengths were very high because of the large amount of enamel bonding available, the feldspathic materials used at the time had strength limitations. Now, because new materials such as lithium disilicate are available at minimal thickness, there is a resurgence of preparationless or minimal preparation options. This resurgence has created a positive effect on the profession as a whole and serves to reeducate the patients and profession to the important philosophy that minimal removal of existing tooth structure should always be a top priority.

TEMPORIZATION

One of the key concepts that dentist's need to understand is that provisionals serve as the foundation to building a successful case. The 2 most common methods to creating provisionals are using templates from a direct mock-up technique or laboratory wax-up. With a direct mock-up, the restoring dentist uses a flowable composite to add directly to the patients existing dentition creating an ideal smile. Once this mock-up is completed, the dentist makes an impression and uses this as a guide for the final

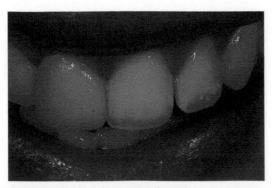

Fig. 9. Clear incisal character displayed on natural tooth.

temporaries. Another option would be to have the laboratory create a wax-up idealizing the patients existing tooth form. This wax-up is then used to create a matrix for provisional fabrication. Although the methods differ in technique, the result is that patients have a set of provisionals that they can wear while the final porcelain is created. Any functional or aesthetic issues can be worked out with plastic instead of the final porcelain, thus allowing patients to approve their provisional smile before insertion of the final porcelain. Careful planning and attention to provisionals are essential for predictable outcomes and satisfied patients.

CASE PRESENTATION

When the patient first arrived to the office, it was immediately apparent that he was wearing down his anterior teeth. As a recent college graduate, he thought that having a better smile might help him be competitive in the job market. A recent survey by the AACD revealed that a person with a pleasing smile is more likely to get hired for a job (**Figs. 10** and **11**). A photograph of lips in repose or at rest showed minimal, if any, tooth display, with the central incisors measuring only 9 mm (**Fig. 12**). The first step was to prepare a mock-up ideal incisal edge position for teeth 8 and 9 using flowable composite. By starting with the central incisors, the dentist can develop the rest of the smile and the patient can visualize the intended result (**Fig. 13**). Photographs are made along with reduction guides and impression template for final provisionals before removing the mock-up. After consultation with the laboratory technician regarding the materials, it was decided that a thin application of lithium dislicate veneer would satisfy the restorative demands. Careful preparations were completed with diamond instruments while constantly referring to reduction guides to confirm that the preparations stay within the enamel layer while ensuring a passive fit that is devoid of any sharp angles.

The Lava Chairside Oral Scanner C.O.S., 3M ESPE (3M ESPE Division, St Paul, MN, USA), was used to accurately capture digital impressions of the preparations and opposing arch along the centric occlusion bite record (**Fig. 14**). The prescription was filled out on the screen and the case e-mailed for processing. It takes about 3 days for the mounted, articulated, pinned models to arrive in the laboratory. The first step for the ceramist, after viewing the preparations, is to confirm the horizontal reference. As mentioned earlier, a midline cant will most often be noticed by even the most nondentally educated person, whereas a midline deviation will often go unnoticed. In general, a laboratory technician should mount the study casts in the same relation as

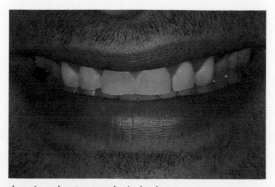

Fig. 10. Smile view showing short worn incisal edges.

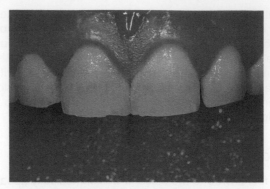

Fig. 11. Close-up view shows severely worn incisal edges.

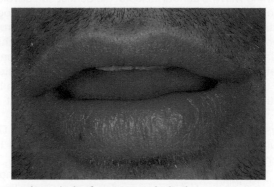

Fig. 12. Lips in repose shows lack of proper tooth display.

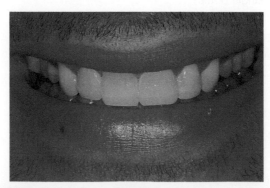

Fig. 13. Mock-up of incisal edges shows improved smile line.

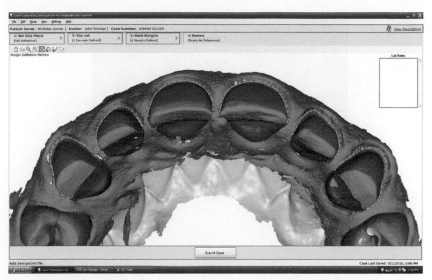

Fig. 14. Digital impression image from the Lava Chairside Oral Scanner C.O.S.

a photograph of the patient with the provisionals. This mounting should be compared with the stick bite as well. Once the case is properly mounted, fabrication of the ceramics can begin.

During the process of fabricating the case, the ceramist will often compare the porcelain shapes with those of the provisionals, original teeth, as well as photographs. By fabricating a matrix of the incisal edge positions of the temporaries, one is able to confirm that the porcelain design follows the patient-approved provisional created by the doctor (**Fig. 15**). The porcelain is layered in several steps to achieve the desired hue, value, chroma, and incisal character or halo effect. On completion of the ceramic, the technician etches the internal surface with the proper hydrofluoric acid so that they are ready for resin bonding.

On the day of insertion, the provisionals are carefully removed and the preparations cleaned and disinfected. For this patient, no anesthesia was used because the preparations were completely in enamel and the patient experienced zero sensitivity even after etching (**Fig. 16**). A dry try-in was performed to confirm the marginal and proximal fit (**Fig. 17**). Typical "total etch" porcelain to enamel bonding was accomplished using a fifth generation single bottle system (Adper Single Bond Plus Adhesive and RelyX

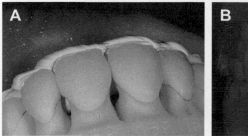
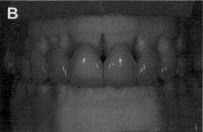

Fig. 15. (*A*) Incisal edge guide from the provisional provides a reference for the lab. (*B*) Restorations showing proper contours and color distribution.

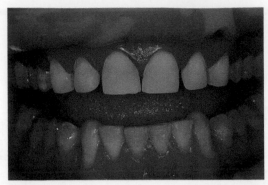

Fig. 16. Etched preparations showing significant enamel bonding available.

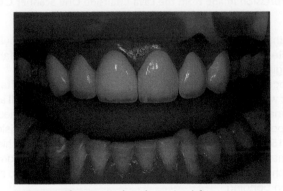

Fig. 17. Dry try-in used to verify marginal and proximal fit.

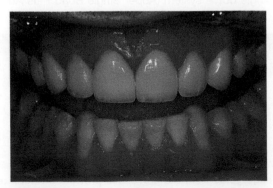

Fig. 18. Immediate postseating.

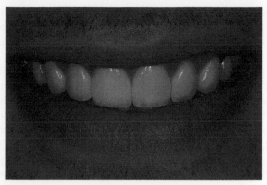

Fig. 19. Improved smile line and natural aesthetics.

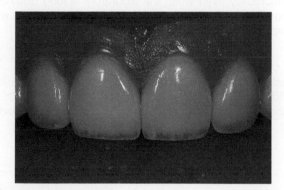

Fig. 20. Detail of incisal edge porcelain.

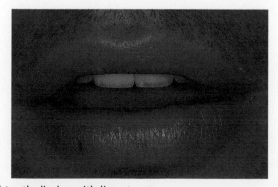

Fig. 21. Improved tooth display with lips at rest.

Transleucent Veneer Cement, 3M ESPE, 3M ESPE Division, St Paul, MN, USA). A rapid seating technique was used, and all restorations were seated, tacked, and cement cleaned followed by final curing for 40 seconds with an oxygen barrier of glycerin gel.

Gentle cleaning at the margins was completed with a No. 12 Bard Parker (BP) blade (Bard Parker, Franklin Lakes, NJ, USA); no burs were used on the facial margins. Lingual margins were finished with a fine red stripe football diamond (Brassler, Savannah, GA, USA) and polished after occlusion verification using Shofu rubber tips (Shofu Dental Inc, San Marcos, CA, USA), medium and fine. Interproximal areas were cleaned and polished using a yellow perforated diamond strip, Brasseler, and floss passed through to verify the interproximal cleanliness (see **Fig. 17**).

This case was finished with minor occlusal equilibration, addition of composite to lower canines, and full coverage bite guard therapy for nighttime use.

The final photographs of this case reveal the kind of results that can be achieved routinely by following proven systems and techniques. Having a clear understanding of the goals of a case and being able to communicate accurately with the ceramist are the keys to success. By using digital cameras and digital impression technology, we are able to improve our ability to not only communicate but also enhance outcomes and improve predictability even when the laboratory is long distance. This case is an example of how proper planning and communication produce excellent clinical results while improving function and aesthetics (**Figs. 18–21**).

REFERENCE

1. American Academy of Cosmetic Dentistry. Can a new smile make you appear more successful and intelligent? Madison (WI): The Academy; 2010. Available from: http://www.aacd.com/index.php?module=cms&page=75. Accessed January 25, 2011.

Soft and Hard Tissue Management Using Lasers in Esthetic Restoration

Hugh D. Flax, DDS[a,b],*

KEYWORDS

- Lasers • Cosmetic dentistry • Minimally invasive
- Closed flap gum lifts

Laser technology has become preeminent in the evolution of appearance enhancements. Dentistry has seen a huge breakthrough with the introduction of a combination hard-soft tissue erbium wavelength. The conservative nature of this technique has created a firm footing in the antiaging trend that is spanning the globe. Among the many benefits of this technique are less invasive care and quicker healing responses. Furthermore, these techniques can allow a cosmetic dentist to control gingival and osseous contours with added artistry in the pursuit of esthetic dental principles and more efficient use of patient time; thus raising customer service experiences.

In this article, conservative laser and cosmetic modalities are discussed that allows a clinician to be more comfortable in buying a soft/hard tissue laser and also to more quickly become adept with implementing these techniques.

HISTORICAL LASER BACKGROUND

In 1960, Theodore Maiman, a scientist with Hughes Aircraft Corporation, developed the first working laser, emitting energy from a ruby crystal. This same technology was applied to teeth by Dr Leon Goldman in 1965, causing painless surface crazing of enamel. In the 1970s and 1980s, researchers attempted using other media, such as CO_2 (wavelength 10,600 nm), to better treat soft and hard dental structures. In 1987, the Food and Drug Administration (FDA) approved Myers and Myers' Nd:YAG

The author has nothing to disclose.
Case reports 1 and 2 are reprinted from The Journal of Cosmetic Dentistry, 2010 American Academy of Cosmetic Dentistry, All rights reserved, www.aacd.com; with permission.
[a] American Academy of Cosmetic Dentistry, 402 West Wilson Street, Madison, WI 53703, USA
[b] Private Practice, Atlanta, GA, USA
* 1100 Lake Hearn Drive, Suite 440, Atlanta, GA 30342.
E-mail address: h.flax@FlaxDental.com

Dent Clin N Am 55 (2011) 383–402
doi:10.1016/j.cden.2011.01.008
0011-8532/11/$ – see front matter © 2011 Elsevier Inc. All rights reserved.

laser for commercial purposes to treat dental soft tissues.[1] Three years later, the Kavo Key Laser (Kaltenbach and Voight GmbH and Co, Biberach/ Ris, Germany) introduced successful hard tissue treatment to German dentistry using an erbium:yttrium-aluminium-garnet system (ER:YAG, wavelength 2940 nm). It was not until 1997 that the FDA cleared use of this breakthrough in the United States for caries removal, cavity preparation, and tooth conditioning. With the introduction of the ErCr:YSGG wavelength (erbium, chromium: yttrium-scandium-gallium-garnet, 2780 nm), dentists had the ability to precisely alter bone and dental hard tissues, as well as perform some minor soft tissue modifications.[2] A visual perspective of the many choices in laser wavelengths is shown in **Fig. 1**.

BIOLOGIC MECHANISMS AND ADVANTAGES OF LASERS

Laser light can have many interactions with their target tissues. Because dental tissues have complex compositions, the light is affected by the pigmentation and water content, as well as the wavelength and mode of emission of the light. As a rule of thumb, wavelengths 1000 nm or shorter are well absorbed by darker tissues and hemoglobin. Furthermore, those wavelengths longer than 1000 nm tend to interact well with water and hydroxyapatite, found in bone and tooth structures. **Table 1** summarizes this wavelength absorption. It is important to remember that although therapeutic effects are optimized by following these characteristics, the critical issues in treatment are how easily the light can be delivered to the tissue, any potential for necrosis, and the goals of treatment.

The advantages of lasers when properly used by well-trained clinicians (who understand physics in laser usage) are the following[3]:

- Ability to seal blood vessels, creating a more bloodless field and decreased need for sutures
- Seal lymphatic vessels, decreasing postoperative swelling and scarring
- Reduced mechanical trauma
- Instant sterilization of the surgical site that can be helpful in operative procedures and surgical care, including implant placement and rescue[4]

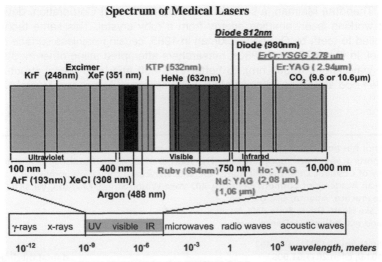

Fig. 1. Full spectrum of wavelengths in the medical field.

Table 1		
Wavelength absorption characteristics of dental lasers		
Laser	Wavelength (nm)	Absorbant
Alexandrite (2x)	377	Calculus
Argon	488 & 515	Hemoglobin, melanin, resin catalyst
HeNe	632	Melanin
Diode	810–980	Melanin, water
Nd:YAG	1064	Melanin, water, dentin
Ho:YAG	2120	Water, dentin
ErCr:YSGG	2780	Water, hydroxyapatite
Er:YAG	2940	Water, hydroxyapatite
CO_2	10,600	Hydroxyapatite, water

- Reduced bacteremia
- Minimal postoperative discomfort.

Taking advantage of these benefits is huge clinically. Furthermore, patients prosper from decreased fears of discomfort and postprocedure complications, and the added precision minimizes the invasiveness of procedures. Undoubtedly, these advantages clearly improve the perception and marketability of a dental practice, both by retaining and attracting patients and staff.

The mechanism of action for laser treatment of hard tissues with erbium lasers is the rapid subsurface expansion of the interstitially trapped water within the mineral substrate that causes a massive volume expansion leading to microexplosions in the surrounding tissues. Using water coolant and short pulse duration minimizes the heat transfer to the tooth.[2,5] Soft tissue procedures, such as incision, contouring, ablation, and hemostasis, are performed better at other wavelengths, such as that emitted by the diode (wavelength 812–980 nm). However, by adjusting the power density (the relationship of the wattage and focal distance of the laser beam, defined as W/cm^2), erbium lasers can still be used as a multipurpose modality with same microexplosion mechanism as hard tissue. The difference is that there is more of a "shaving" or "planning" of soft tissue than the deeper absorbed dedicated soft tissue laser.[6]

Although lasers are less traumatic and more comfortable, it has also been found that the application to tooth structure has allowed "radiation scattered in enamel and dentin to be entrapped by these natural waveguides and transported to the pulp chamber."[7] It has been postulated that there is a shift in pain fiber sensitivity with a reduction in the action of the sodium-potassium pump at the cellular level, thereby slowing or even stopping nerve conduction in the pulpal tissues long enough to more comfortably ablate enamel and dentin without the use of anesthesia in most cases.[8] Furthermore, Glockner and colleagues[9] reported a decrease in pulpal temperature and thermal damage from 37°C to between 25°C and 30°C after a few seconds of erbium laser exposure.

One area of great debate is the reported increase in bond strengths when using erbium lasers as a result of the microcratering of enamel and dentin.[10,11] Although the roughening of the surface may increase the surface area and physical retention, it is still prudent to continue chemical etching until definitive studies are conclusive.

CAVITY TREATMENT WITH LASERS

Because of the aforementioned advantages of the laser modality, treatment of carious lesions is improved. Using conservative microdentistry principles formulated by

Knight[12] and Millicich and Rainey,[13] it is important to follow a risk management protocol advocated by CAMBRA (CAries Management By Risk Assessment)[14] as follows:

- Diagnose before treatment using DIAGNOdent (KaVo Dental, Charlotte, NC, USA) readings and magnification to visualize risky anatomy, as well as perform CariFree (Oral BioTech, Albany, OR, USA) testing and treatment to help remineralize and possibly reverse suspicious borderline lesions that are close to the threshold measurement of 20.[15]
- Make treatment decisions based on risk.
- Use caries detection die when appropriate so that defective hard tissue is selectively removed by lasers or air abrasion, and preserve the peripheral rim of enamel (**Fig. 2**).
- A sandwich technique that uses glass ionomer composites (GICs) is advantageous to give a predictable seal because of minimized shrinkage and a remineralization effect when restoring decayed lesions (**Fig. 3**).

After managing the patient's expectations for care (ie, discussing the laser experience), an Isolite (Isolite Systems, Santa Barbara, CA) is applied to improve isolation in a comfortable manner. A ninety second "laser analgesia" application is performed with laser tip (usually a 600 μm glass quartz tip) defocused from and perpendicular to the enamel surface at a height of 10 mm, with a setting 4.5 W, 60% water, 30% air. When the analgesia cycle is completed, the laser tip is brought with a 0.5–1.0 mm of the enamel and pointed at a buccal or lingual angle parallel to the enamel rods to improve cutting efficiency on the occlusal surface (a perpendicular approach works fine on smooth surface lesions, **Fig. 4**). Carefully dissecting and ablating the decalcified and carious areas along the grooves and trying to preserve the triangular ridges, the enamel is cleansed at this setting, while the less mineralized, more carious dentin is ablated at 3.5 W, 60% water, 30% air. Since the laser tip is only end cutting, any small areas undermining enamel can be removed with spoons or a sharp slow speed round bur, that patient tends not to object. Any white "cratering" caused on the cavosurface or esthetic areas should be smoothed with a medium diamond to avoid any shine through in the future bonding. When the decay is removed, the tooth is restored using a "closed sandwich technique"-with the GIC sealing/replacing the dentin and protected from oral fluids by composite that is acting as an enamel replacement.[16] Composite materials are chosen based on the remaining tooth

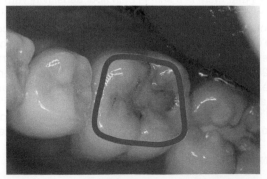

Fig. 2. The peripheral rim of enamel (*red*) acts like a bicycle rim to maintain biomechanical strength of the tooth, where the triangular ridges act like the spokes.

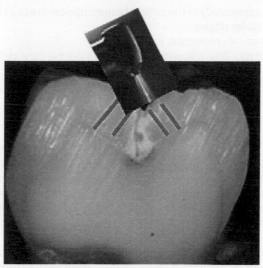

Fig. 3. Treatment of the occlusal decay with a laser. Unlike typical operative approaches to breaking through the enamel "roof" over the decalcified enamel and dentin, the laser cuts more efficiently by using an angulation parallel to the enamel rods versus the standard perpendicular to the enamel surface. Smooth surface caries can be treated in a more customary manner.

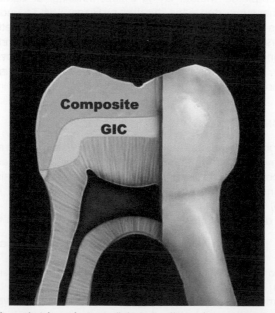

Fig. 4. The closed sandwich technique (labeled) allows for a decreased polymerization shrinkage and direction remineralization of the dentin by glass ionomer.

structure available, particularly in the critical biomechanical areas of the peripheral rim of enamel and triangular ridges.

A video (MMC 1) of this technique is provided.

Supplementary data. The following are the Supplementary data related to this article:

Supplementary data related to this article can be found online at doi: 10.1016/j. cden.2011.01.008.

LASER COSMETIC SMILE ENHANCEMENT

Charles Darwin said that "Beauty is the association of many complex associations." Undoubtedly, this theory can be applied to the art and science of esthetic dentistry. Harmony of function, biology, and appearance is paramount in creating long-term results for patients. Fortunately, the efforts of many pioneers such as Pankey and Mann,[17] Dawson,[18] and Lee[19] have allowed contemporaries to achieve bioesthetic results more predictably.

One of the more challenging aspects of these multiple associations is gingival symmetry and health. Rufenacht[20] and Chiche[21] have detailed the artistic components (contours, proportions) of a memorable smile. Dolt and Robbins[22] describe a differential diagnostic process for recognizing, diagnosing, and treating esthetic dilemmas in gingival/tooth architecture. The classic study by Kois[23] defined the anatomic relationships of the dentogingival complex (DGC). Maintaining biologic width is predictable when measured clinically at 3 mm direct facially and at 3 mm to 5 mm interproximally from the free gingival margin to the osseous crest. Ultimately, the gingival margin must mimic the osseous curvatures to maintain a healthy gingival restorative interface.

The study by Wang[24] showed that osseous crown lengthening with ErCr:YSGG laser could be completed without laying a flap, suturing, or damaging the bone. This finding is further supported in the literature by Rizoiu[25] who found that the thermal coagulative results and ablation qualities were similar to those created by a dental bur. From a patient perspective, the decreased need for suturing and shorter healing times should definitely increase case acceptance to complement the growing demand for esthetic dentistry. In addition, the restorative dentist can have increased artistic control of the periodontal framework.

SMILE DESIGN CONSIDERATIONS

There are many books and articles that cover this topic well. Calamia and colleagues[26] have created an evaluation form that covers the details in a systematic and thorough manner for data collection and diagnostic planning. Furthermore, using the American Academy of Cosmetic Dentistry series of photography is critical for collaborative planning[27] (Fig. 5).[26]

Although smile design is subjective, these are some key areas to focus on:

- The golden proportion of anterior teeth from canine to canine should be considered.
- The width to length ratio of central incisors should be considered. Because the centrals are the main starting point for smile design, the incisal edge position is most critical in facially generated planning. However, if they are too square or elongated, the disproportion can disrupt the esthetics of a smile. The recommended width to length ratio is 0.75:0.80. If a periodontal

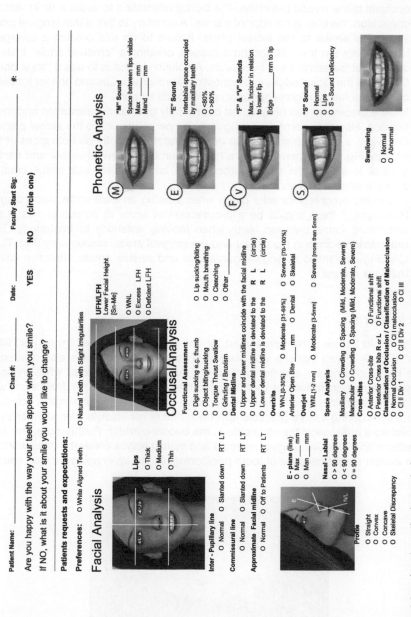

NYU College of Dentistry Smile Evaluation Form

Patient Name: _____ Chart #: _____ Date: _____ Faculty Start Sig: _____ #: _____

Are you happy with the way your teeth appear when you smile?   YES   NO   (circle one)

If NO, what is it about your smile you would like to change? _____

Patients requests and expectations:

Preferences: O White Aligned Teeth   O Natural Teeth with Slight Irregularities

Facial Analysis

Lips
O Thick
O Medium
O Thin

Inter - Pupillary line
O Normal   O Slanted down   RT   LT

Commissural line
O Normal   O Slanted down   RT   LT

Approximate Facial midline
O Normal   O Off to Patients   RT   LT

E - plane (line)
O Max _____ mm
O Man _____ mm

Nasal - Labial
O > 90 degrees
O < 90 degrees
O = 90 degrees

Profile
O Straight
O Convex
O Concave
O Skeletal Discrepancy

Occlusal Analysis

UFH/LFH
Lower Facial Height
[Sn-Me]
O WNL
O Excess   LFH
O Deficient LFH

Functional Assessment
O Digit sucking e.g. thumb
O Object biting/sucking
O Tongue Thrust Swallow
O Grinding / Bruxism

O Lip sucking/biting
O Mouth breathing
O Clenching
O Other _____

Dental Midline
O Upper and lower midlines coincide with the facial midline
O Upper dental midline is deviated to the   R   L   (circle)
O Lower dental midline is deviated to the   R   L   (circle)

Overbite
O WNL-[0-30%]   O Moderate [31-69%]   O Severe [70-100%]
Anterior Open Bite _____ mm   O Dental   O Skeletal

Overjet
O WNL-[1-2 mm]   O Moderate [3-5mm]   O Severe [more than 5mm]

Space Analysis
Maxillary   O Crowding O Spacing (Mild, Moderate, Severe)
Mandibular O Crowding O Spacing (Mild, Moderate, Severe)

Cross-bites
O Anterior Cross-bite   O Functional shift
O Posterior Cross bite R or L   O Functional shift
Classification of Occlusion / Classification of Malocclusion
O Normal Occlusion   O CI I malocclusion
O CI I Div 1   O CI II Div 1   O CI II Div 2   O CI III

Phonetic Analysis

"M" Sound
Space between lips visible
Max _____ mm
Mand _____ mm

"E" Sound
Interlabial space occupied
by maxillary teeth
O <80%
O >80%

"F" & "V" Sounds
Max. Incisor in relation
to lower lip
Edge _____ mm to lip

"S" Sound
O Normal
O Lips
O S - Sound Deficiency

Swallowing
O Normal
O Abnormal

Fig. 5. Organizing data in smile design helps improve predictability in the final result, as well as document information medicolegally when dealing with subjective outcomes. To avail this form, e-mail Dr John R. Calamia at jrc1@nyu.edu.

solution is appropriate, erbium laser treatment allows for soft and hard tissue adjustments in proportion.

- The incisal plane is ideally suited to a horizontal orientation, often parallel to the interpupillary line (unless the eyes are canted). The edges should also follow a curve created by a symmetrically curved lower lip. Furthermore, the posterior occlusal plane should blend into the incisal orientation to avoid a tilt in vertical orientation, the buccal corridor of a smile. A corollary to this is that gingival plane should be similar to the incisal plane. Failure to do this creates a divergent tension between the soft and hard tissues, creating a "crooked smile" instead of one that is beautiful and believable. A solution to this is to use 2 "stick bites" that orient the incisal edges in diagnostic planning/wax-ups and one for focusing on gingival height alignment during periodontal surgery.
- Midline placement can be affected horizontally by skeletal orientation and tooth position. However, vertical canting must be perpendicular to the incisal plane.
- Gingivally, a more attractive smile demonstrates symmetry on both sides of the midline (**Fig. 6**). Furthermore, as a rule of thumb, the central incisor and canine gingival levels are the same, although the lateral incisor soft tissue crest is approximately 1 mm shorter.
- Geometric progressions take place when viewing an ideal smile. According to Rufenacht,[20] there should be a progression of acute to obtuse angles in the embrasure forms between teeth when moving anteriorly to posteriorly. This progression occurs in the incisal and the gingival areas, respectively (**Fig. 7**).
- Creating similarities in gingival curvatures and zeniths create attractive smiles that look natural.

CASE REPORT 1

A 38-year-old female patient presented for correction of what she termed her "tilted smile" (**Fig. 8**). Given that she was starting a new sales career, she also desired to make her teeth brighter and the smile much broader. Furthermore, while trying to balance the responsibilities of motherhood, the patient shared her frustration with previous dental consultations that focused only on orthodontic or surgical solutions without considering a more practical approach that fit her lifestyle. Her smile analysis established a collapse of the bicuspids in the buccal corridor. Furthermore, the axial inclinations and irregular gingival margins and incisal edges created a downward tilt to the patient's right because of tooth positioning. Close-up imaging showed healthy

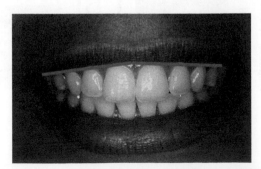

Fig. 6. Gingival symmetry from a labial view. Notice that the plane follows the curvature of the upper lip.

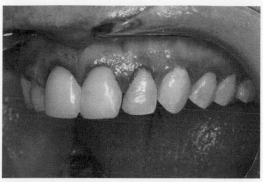

Fig. 7. A geometric progression from acute to obtuse angles occurring in the incisal and gingival embrasures in a smile when following the teeth in an anterior-posterior direction. This architecture was created immediately after laser sculpting of the soft tissue before adjusting the osseous contour via a closed flap approach.

gingival tissues as well as a weakened right central incisor from a large composite (**Fig. 9**).

Full clinical examination with radiographs and mounted models revealed the following:

- Biomechanically, most of the patient's teeth remained strong because of previously received dental care.
- The periodontal condition of the soft and hard tissues was healthy.
- Occlusally, load testing was normal (after muscle relaxation) and there was obvious centric relation–centric occlusion anterior-vertical slide because of a premature contact at tooth number 30.
- Esthetically, the width-length ratio of upper centrals was 1.20, far from the ideal range of 0.75 to 1.00. Tooth shade was a Vita A2.

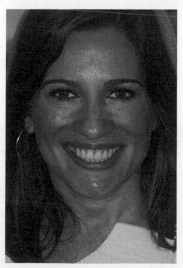

Fig. 8. Visualizing the entire oral-facial composition helps diagnose the less harmonious features of the smile.

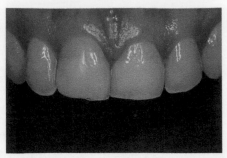

Fig. 9. Close-up photography is essential to planning periorestorative care.

Given the patient's previous history and her desire for minimally invasive dental care, a conservative strategy was devised that allows the correction of the problems and causes in a multitasking manner:

- Muscle and bite therapy with a Tanner appliance followed by careful equilibration aided by the T-scan (Tekscan System, South Boston, MA, USA)
- Three-dimensional wax-up using a Stratos articulator (Ivoclar-Vivadent, Amherst, NY, USA) **Fig. 10**
- Home bleaching of the lower teeth with Opalescence 15% (Ultradent, South Jordan, UT, USA)
- Closed-flap periodontal modification with the Waterlase ErCr:YSGG (Biolase Technology, San Clemente, CA, USA) while the first 3 items were being accomplished. The combination of these 4 steps allowed to save time and also to carefully monitor the progress on a weekly basis
- Definitive restorative care with porcelain veneers and a crown on tooth number 8.

At the initial closed periodontal lift, the ErCr:YSGG laser was used in 3 modes (ie, gingival sculpting, osseous recontouring, and biostimulation). Before anesthesia, the desired framework was planned and outlined using a fine marker (**Fig. 11**). Furthermore, a stick bite was used to not only establish an ideal incisal plane but also properly align the gingival margins (**Fig. 12**).

With the settings of 2 W, 20 pulses per second, 20% air, and 20% water, a G-6 tip (600 μm in diameter) was used to shape the labial gingival region. No tissue necrosis or significant bleeding occurred as a result of using the laser's relatively lower settings.

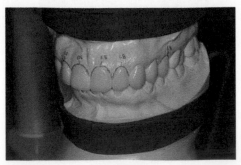

Fig. 10. A mounted diagnostic wax-up is a critical road map to planning a realistic result.

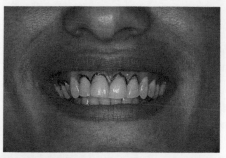

Fig. 11. Outlining the desired gingival margins, before anesthesia, communicates a blueprint to the patient and restorative team.

All areas were "sounded" using a periodontal probe (**Fig. 13**). At the facial margins, osseous sculpting required great precision to maintain a 3-mm DGC. A specially tapered T4 tip (400 micrometers in diameter) was used at a 25% higher wattage of 2.5 W. Before usage, the tip was measured and marked to 3 mm to maintain controlled adjustments within the gingival sulcus during periodontal probing movement of the tip (**Fig. 14**). The resection was smoothed with a 7/8 curette (**Fig. 15**). Using low-level laser therapy, at a setting of 0.25 W, a decrease in the release of inflammatory histamine and increased fibroblasts for junctional epithelial growth was achieved by "frosting" the outer epithelium and injection sites (**Fig. 16**). There was immediate improvement of the geometric progression of gingival embrasures. The patient was placed on a vigorous homecare regimen (Oxygel; Oxyfresh, Coeur d'Alene, ID, USA) and closely monitored for a month while occlusal therapy and bleaching procedures were performed.

Four weeks postsurgically, the tissues were healed and restorative care could be initiated. The patient's teeth were prepared for veneers and a crown with mild soft tissue reshaping to fine-tune the previous treatment. After impressions and bite registrations, prototype provisionals (eg, Luxatemp Plus; Zenith DMG, Englewood, NJ, USA) were fabricated using the "shrink-wrap" technique.

The patient was sent home with the same home care regimen and to "test-drive" her new smile for esthetics and function. She returned in a week to perfect the prototype's occlusion, color, and morphology. Photos and models were sent to the laboratory providing a final blueprint for the porcelain restorations (**Fig. 17**).

Four weeks later, the provisionals and cement were carefully removed from the teeth. All restorations were tried in individually and as a group to verify fit and esthetics.

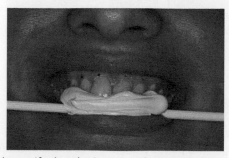

Fig. 12. A stick bite helps verify that the incisal and gingival planes are parallel.

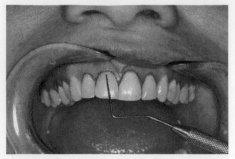

Fig. 13. Sounding to bone after atraumatic soft tissue sculpting.

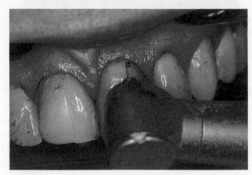

Fig. 14. To modify the bone, a very tight up and down movement is performed using the black mark as a reference after the gingival scallop.

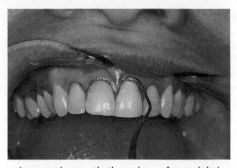

Fig. 15. A curette helps clean and smooth the sulcus of any debris.

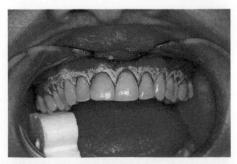

Fig. 16. A "laser bandage" was placed along the area of treatment to improve the healing time and decrease patient discomfort.

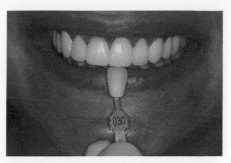

Fig. 17. Detailed information helps the laboratory translate clinical results to the porcelain restorations.

After the patient's enthusiastic approval, the porcelain was bonded using the 2 × 2 technique and isolation. Margins were smoothed and polished, and occlusion was balanced with the T-scan. A protective nighttime appliance was created to add longevity to the rehabilitation. The patient felt that the results exceeded her expectations (**Figs. 18** and **19**).

Use of a hard/soft tissue laser is a wonderful adjunctive tool for cosmetic and restorative dentistry. The above case demonstrates that this type of laser technology gives dentists the ability to make significant soft and hard tissue changes while being minimally invasive. These changes not only improve the final esthetic outcome of the case but also provide the physiologic functional parameters required for successful dentistry.

CASE REPORT 2

A 62-year-old female patient presented for correction of what she termed her "Spongebob smile" (**Figs. 20** and **21**). Clinical photographs demonstrated how

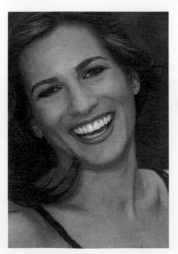

Fig. 18. Great improvement in esthetics boosted this patient's self-confidence and pride in her dental care.

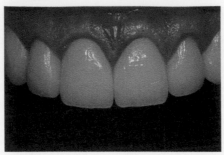

Fig. 19. Ideal proportions and emergence profiles create long-term healthy tissues and bioesthetics.

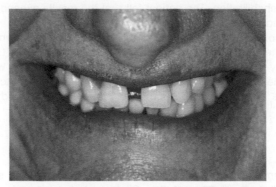

Fig. 20. The large midline was a major detriment to this patient's appearance.

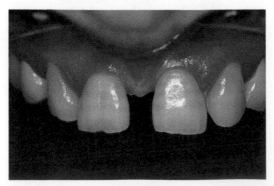

Fig. 21. Broad widths of the gingival papillae created an unfavorable framework to create more harmonious esthetics.

self-conscious the patient was about her smile's appearance. A large midline diastema that measured approximately 4 mm was the centerpiece of a dentition that had missing maxillary canines and discolored metal-ceramic restorations that had been placed without a master plan for complete dental health and appearance. Consequently, the patient was frustrated that her previous care would prevent her from achieving an improved smile. Further challenges included the presence of a deep overbite and a thick deep labial frenum. Other considerations were budgeting and time constraints, as well as a desire to use a conservative approach.

Diastema closure is an art form that involves not only the repositioning of proximal surfaces but also integrating the gingival interface and occlusion to create ideal proportions and natural contours that can be easily cleansed. Specialty referral was ruled out by the patient because of the aforementioned concerns. A plan was, therefore, devised to laser sculpt the soft and hard tissue to create an external framework to train the gingival (first stage) and eventually place porcelain restorations from teeth number 4 through teeth number 14 (second stage). These new contours would be determined with the aid of a mounted diagnostic wax-up (**Fig. 22**). Because the patient's time was at a minimum, whitening and occlusal procedures were also performed during the first stage of periodontal-restorative procedures.

At the initial closed periodontal lift, a Waterlase ErCr:YSGG laser was used in 3 modes (ie, gingival sculpting, osseous recontouring and smoothing, and frenectomy). The desired framework was planned and outlined using a fine marker, and a G-6 tip was subsequently used to shape the gingival region. No tissue necrosis or significant bleeding occurred as a result of using the laser's relatively lower settings. A flowable composite was then cemented along the mesial aspects of teeth numbers 8 and 9. After smoothing with a "safe end" bur (H135TDF; Axis Dental, Irving, TX, USA), a solid matrix was created to mold the midline papilla (**Fig. 23**). Osseous sculpting required great precision to maintain a 3-mm DGC. A specially tapered T4 tip was used at a higher wattage of 2.5 W. Before usage, the tip was measured and marked to 3 mm to maintain controlled adjustments within the gingival sulcus during a machine stitch movement of the tip. The resection was smoothed with a 7/8 curette. The frenectomy was cleanly performed at the soft tissue setting, causing a release of the midline papilla and great freedom of the upper lip (**Fig. 24**). At a setting of 0.25 W, biostimulation of the outer epithelium helped to decrease the release of histamine and increased fibroblasts for junctional epithelial growth. The patient was placed on a vigorous homecare regimen (Oxygel) and closely monitored for a month while occlusal therapy procedures were performed.

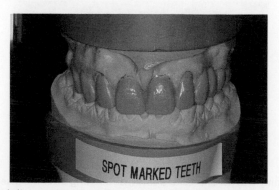

Fig. 22. A mounted diagnostic wax-up is a critical road map to planning a realistic result.

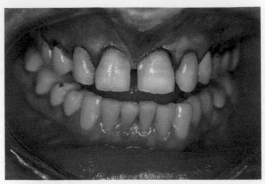

Fig. 23. After the soft tissue was laser sculpted, flowable composite was placed and polished to train the contour of the proximal surfaces of the midline papilla.

At 4 weeks postoperatively, the tissues were healed and restorative care was initiated. Using the diagnostic wax-up as a guide, the width of the midline papilla was determined and modified horizontally to match the blueprint (**Figs. 25** and **26**). The patient's teeth were prepared for veneers/crowns, and mild soft tissue reshaping was performed. After impressions and bite registrations, prototype provisionals (Luxatemp Plus) were fabricated. Improvement and acute angles for the papillae, which are a reflection of the ideal geometric esthetic progression from anterior to posterior, are observed (**Fig. 27**).

The patient was provisionalized for 30 days. Minimal modifications were necessary to improve the patient's appearance and bite. Measurements and photos were sent to the ceramist. Using the temporary model, a labioincisal matrix was created to maintain a consistent aesthetic and functional relationship (**Fig. 28**).

The restorations were returned from the laboratory preetched and silanated. They were inspected for contour and fit not only labially for aesthetics but also occlusally for hygiene purposes (**Fig. 29**). Using isolation procedures, the Authentic porcelain (Microstar Dental, Lawrenceville, GA, USA) was bonded using translucent resin cement (eg, Variolink II, Ivoclar Vivadent, Amherst, NY, USA). The patient was ecstatic about the aesthetic results achieved through the periorestorative procedure (**Figs. 30** and **31**).

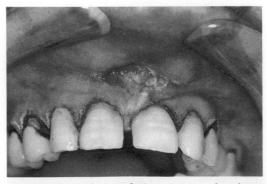

Fig. 24. A frenectomy was performed at a soft tissue setting after the osseous sculpting was completed. Note the minimal trauma and bleeding after use of the laser.

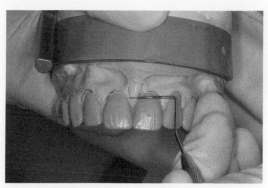

Fig. 25. The width of the midline papilla is critical to achieving the planned geometric progression from anterior to posterior teeth.

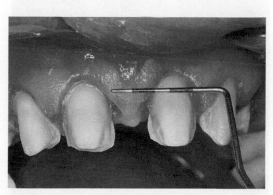

Fig. 26. The midline papilla is checked intraorally. Note that the margins are placed subgingivally to optimize the emergence profile of the porcelain.

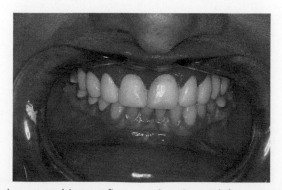

Fig. 27. Provisionals are test-driven to fine-tune function and the patient's esthetic desires.

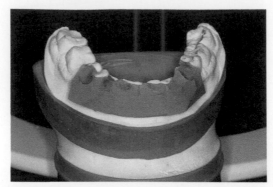

Fig. 28. Mounting of the approved prototypes allows the laboratory to create a labial incisal silicon matrix.

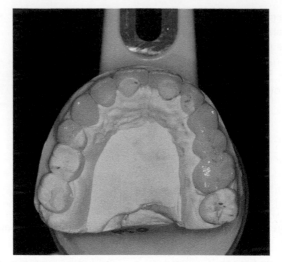

Fig. 29. Natural incisal thicknesses and proximal embrasures promote better function and health.

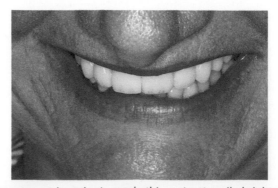

Fig. 30. Great improvement in esthetics made this patient's smile brighter.

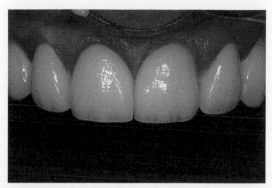

Fig. 31. A beautiful and believe smile created in a nontraditional but predictable manner.

SUMMARY

With expanding emphasis on minimally invasive care (eg, Botox, mesotherapy), dentistry has as amazing an ally in laser technology. The literature demonstrating the health benefits is being augmented with the cosmetic advantages as well. Carefully using the hard and soft tissue lasers gives cosmetic dentistry a patient friendly tool to predictably and comfortably compliment the many advances in smile design. These are truly exciting times for patients and professionals alike!

REFERENCES

1. Coluzzi D. Fundamentals of dental lasers: science and instruments. Dent Clin North Am 2004;48:750.
2. Van As G. Erbium lasers in dentistry. Dent Clin North Am 2004;48:1018–9, 1028.
3. Wigdor H, Walsh J, Featherstone J, et al. Lasers in dentistry. Lasers Surg Med 1995;16:103–33.
4. Schwartz F, Rothamel D, Becker J, et al. Influence of an Er: YAG laser on the surface structure of titanium implants. Schweiz Monatsschr Zahnmed 2003; 113(6):660–71 [in French, German].
5. Freiberg RJ, Cozean C. Pulsed erbium laser ablation of hard dental tissue: the effects of atomized water spray versus water surface film. Lasers in dentistry VIII. Proc SPIE 2002;4610:74–84.
6. Bornstein E, Lomke MA. The safety and effectiveness of dental Er: YAG lasers: a literature review with specific reference to bone. Dent Today 2003;22(10): 129–33.
7. Neev J. Modern optics and dentistry. In: Miserdino L, Pick R, editors. Lasers in dentistry. Carol Stream (IL): Quintessence Publishing Co; 1995. p. 287.
8. Hadley J, Young DA, Eversole LR, et al. Laser powered hydrokinetic system for caries removal and cavity preparation. J Am Dent Assoc 2000;131:777–85.
9. Glockner K, Rumpler J, Ebeleseder K, et al. Intrapulpal pressure during preparation with a Er:YAG laser compared to the conventional bur: an in vitro study. Lasers Surg Med 1999;17:153–7.
10. Hibst R. Lasers for caries removal and cavity preparation: state of the art and future directions. J Oral Laser Appl 2002;2:203–12.
11. Apel C, Schafer C, Gutknecht N. Demineralization of Er:YAG and ErCr:YSGG laser-prepared enamel cavities in vitro. Caries Res 2003;37(1):34–7.

12. Knight GM. The co-cured, light-activated glass-ionomer cement-composite resin restoration. Quintessence Int 1994;25(2):97–100.
13. Milicich G, Rainey JT. Clinical presentations of stress distribution in teeth and the significance in operative dentistry. Pract Periodontics Aesthet Dent 2000;12(7): 695–700.
14. Young D, Featherstone J, Roth J, et al. Caries management by risk assessment: implementation guidelines. J Calif Dent Assoc 2007;35(11):799–805.
15. DIAGNOdent training manual, Kavo. Available at: http://www.kavousa.com/Default.aspx?navid=552872&oid=009&lid=Us&rid=552890. Accessed January 25, 2011.
16. Mount G. Clinical requirements for a successful 'sandwich'—dentine to glass ionomer cement to composite resin. Aust Dent J 1989;34(3):259–65.
17. Pankey L, Mann A. Oral rehabilitation. J Prosthet Dent 1960;10:135–62.
18. Dawson P. Evaluation, diagnosis, and treatment of occlusal problems. 2nd edition. St Louis (MO): CV Mosby Co; 1989.
19. Lee R. Esthetics and its relationship to function. In: Rufenacht C, editor. Fundamentals of esthetics. Carol Stream (IL): Quintessence Publishing Co; 1990. p. 140. Chapter 5.
20. Rufenacht CR. Fundamentals of esthetics. Carol Stream (IL): Quintessence Publishing Co; 1990. p. 104–7. Chapter 4.
21. Chiche G. Esthetics of anterior fixed prosthodontics. Carol Stream (IL): Quintessence Publishing Co; 1994.
22. Dolt A, Robbins J. Altered passive eruption: an etiology of short clinical crowns. Quintessence Int 1997;28(6):363.
23. Kois J. Altering gingival levels: the restorative connection. Part I: biologic variables. J Esthet Dent 1994;6:3–9.
24. Wang X. Morphological changes in bovine mandibular bone irradiated by the ErCr: YSGG laser—an in-vitro study. J Clin Laser Med Surg 2002;20(5):245–50.
25. Rizoiu IR, Eversole L, Kimmel A, et al. Effects of an erbium, chromium: yttrium, scandium, gallium, garnet laser on mucotaneous soft tissues. Oral Surg Oral Med Oral Pathol Oral Radiol Enclod 1996;82:386–95.
26. Calamia J, Levine J, Lipp M. NYU College of Dentistry Smile Evaluation Form (Adapted from the work of Leonard Abrams, 255 South Seventeenth Street, Philadelphia, PA 19103 1987 and Dr. Mauro Fradeani Esthetic Rehabilitation in Fixed Prosthodontics Quintessence Publishing Co. inc Carol Stream, IL 2004 Jonathan B. Levine, DMD GoSMILEAesthetics 923 5th Avenue, New York, NY 10021).
27. American Academy of Cosmetic Dentistry photo guide. Madison (WI): American Academy of Cosmetic Dentistry; 2009. p. 4–22.

Esthetic and Functional Consideration in Restoring Endodontically Treated Teeth

Richard D. Trushkowsky, DDS*

KEYWORDS

• Endodontics • Ceramic • Post • Restoration

The selection of the best restoration for an endodontically treated tooth in the aesthetic zone[1] depends on strength and the ability to recreate the form, function, and aesthetics of the natural tooth.[2] The increased use of all-ceramic materials is a result of improved ceramic materials and adhesive systems.[3] However, the advent of the current variety of translucent ceramic systems makes the shade of the abutment important in achieving the desired aesthetic outcome. Carossa and colleagues[4] studied different posts and cores and thought that, although there were significant differences spectrophotometrically, clinically these differences were not noticeable. Deger and colleagues,[5] Vichi and colleagues,[6] and Nakamura and colleagues[7] arrived at different conclusions. They found that translucent ceramic crowns thinner than 1.6 mm are affected by the color of the core. Vichi and colleagues[6] found that when the thickness of the ceramic crown was 1 mm, color differences with the adjacent teeth are visually noticeable. Color differences decreased when the thickness was increased to 1.5 mm, and at 2.0 mm, no differences were noticeable. Michalakis and colleagues[8] found that cast posts can result in root discoloration and have a blue-gray effect if the overlying bone and soft tissue are thin, which would be especially important if a high lip line or broad smile exposes the restoration. De Rouffignac and de Cooman[9] suggested using cast metal posts and cores with 2 thin metal tags to retain a ceramic for the core. However, this only addressed the optical effects in the

The author has nothing to disclose.
Department of Cariology and Comprehensive Care, New York University College of Dentistry, 345 East 24th Street, New York, NY 10010, USA
* 483 Jefferson Boulevard Staten Island, NY 10312-2332.
E-mail address: ComposiDoc@aol.com

Dent Clin N Am 55 (2011) 403–410
doi:10.1016/j.cden.2011.01.009
dental.theclinics.com

coronal aspect, not in the root. If cast gold is used for the post and core, Carossa and colleagues[4] found greater luminance with a polished core compared with a matte-finished one.

Because the shade of the final restoration is affected by the color of the abutment, the need for a post and the nature of the post must be considered. Previously, a post was considered necessary for reinforcing an endodontically treated tooth, but most recent studies demonstrate a weakening effect rather than reinforcement.[10] Some clinicians feel that the use of adhesive materials allow the clinician to bond the post to the dentin, the core to the post, and the ultimate restoration to the post-core and remaining tooth structure. Theoretically, when the various components with analogous properties are bonded together, the root can be strengthened, but this theory has not been proved.[11] However, when there is insufficient tooth structure present, full coverage restorations may need a post to provide adequate retention.[12]

NEED FOR A POST

Post preparation may increase the risk of root fracture.[13] Teeth that have been debilitated by trauma, caries, or previous restoration are often those that require endodontic treatment. Endodontic access forms require straight-line entrance and the "crown down" technique requires adequate removal of both coronal and radicular dentin to provide a continuously tapered preparation to the apex. The remaining tooth structure needs to be evaluated on its ability to retain and support the final restoration. The type of post and adhesive system that provides the best strength, reliability, aesthetics, and ease of handling should be selected.[14] Peroz and colleagues[15] formulated a classification of the amount of remaining tooth structure that is related to the remaining walls. Class I has all 4 axial walls remaining and only the access preparation, class II has 1 cavity wall removed and could be either an mesial-occlusal or distal-occlusal. Class III is an mesial-occlusal-distal cavity with 2 remaining walls, and class IV has only 1 remaining wall (either a buccal or lingual). Class V has no remaining walls. Dietschi and colleagues[16] delineated the modifications that occur in dentin composition, physical characteristics, fracture resistance, tooth stiffness, and restorative materials and techniques that would be required to effectively restore an endodontically treated tooth. He also determined that there is a change in not only the water content but also the Young modulus, and proportional limit are modified slightly. There is no resulting decrease in compressive strength and tensile strength.

TYPES OF POSTS

Zirconia posts were introduced by Meyenberg and colleagues[17] in 1993. Prefabricated zirconia posts possess some positive attributes such as high strength to bending forces and good optical properties. However, their use with pressed ceramic or composite resin cores has been problematic because of delamination. One-piece milled zirconia post and core eliminates this dilemma, as there is no interface between the post and core. In addition, the diameters of the posts available limit their use in smaller-diameter teeth such as mandibular incisors, lateral incisors, and maxillary first premolars. Zirconia posts also possess a high modulus of elasticity (200 GPa). Some clinicians think that stiffer posts and cores allow increased support for the final restoration and create a more uniform distribution of stress. Others think that a more flexible post would be more beneficial, as bending under load causes loss of the restoration but allows the root system to be accessible for a new restoration. Micromotion of the post and core may result in failure of the luting cement, coronal leakage, and recurrent decay.[18] Zirconium posts are not recommended for posterior teeth because of the higher occlusal forces. In the anterior region, average forces are 222 N, and posts and cores have to be able to withstand these forces.[19]

Zirconia posts are rigid and hard and may cause disastrous fractures of the root; if the post fractures, it would be extremely difficult to remove. Zirconium oxide ceramics also undergo phase transformation at different temperatures. The addition of yttrium oxide to zirconium oxide creates a partially stabilized ceramic (yttria partially stabilized zirconia [YPSZ]). When a crack is initiated in YPSZ with metastable tetragonal grains, the materials high fracture resistance reduces the chance of the crack propagating. Another potential problem is related to fit. The one-piece zirconium posts may have a passive fit relative to the acrylic resin patterns and after adjusting the posts, although not binding did not fit accurately.

Nonrigid Post Systems

- Carbon fiber
- Glass fiber
- Quartz fiber
- Silicon fiber.

Fiber posts were introduced in 1990 and were made of carbon fiber. The carbon fibers were arranged longitudinally and surrounded by an epoxy matrix. These posts had a modulus of elasticity that was supposed to be close to that of dentin and may provide a more uniform distribution of stress on the remaining root structure. Unfortunately, these posts were radiolucent, and the dark color was detrimental to the shade of ceramic crowns.[6] Although fiber posts possess several advantages, there are also disadvantages. Because the modulus of elasticity and flexural strength are similar to that of dentin, occlusal load may result in flexure, possibly resulting in micromovement and subsequently coronal leakage, caries, and loss of the restoration. The presence of a sufficient ferrule reduces the chance of this occurring.[20] However, debonding of the post has been the main cause of failure of restorations in which the post was utilized. Some studies have indicated that an increased volume of cement around the post, especially at the coronal level, may result in loss of retention. Ideally, a thin, uniform cement layer would be beneficial for retention, which can be achieved only with a well-fitting post. A passive post should not transmit stress to the root. Therefore, the fit of the post and the thickness of the cement layer have to be considered to avoid stress transmission to the root.[21] Because most canals are not circular, the use of a preformed post requires modification of canal anatomy, and often the removal of sound dentin, to accommodate the post. The use of an undersized post increases the cement volume and possibly increases the rate of debonding. The clinician has to make a choice between an anatomic and a preformed post. The restoration with an anatomic post usually requires more than 1 visit. A semidirect procedure allows the fabrication of a more anatomic post. The fabrication of an anatomic post reduces the thickness of the cement layer, which may be beneficial, as debonding is more apt to occur with a substantial layer of cement.[22] Because inadequate post stiffness results in increased deformation of the post and localization of stress, the increased thickness of the anatomic post in the coronal area reduces the chance of marginal failure. Fiber posts also have demonstrated loss of flexural strength when they undergo cyclic loading and thermocycling.

One of the drawbacks with any prefabricated post system is the removal of additional tooth structure to accommodate the post. In addition, a curved canal would preclude use of a conventional post. A novel technique has been suggested to overcome these problems. StickTeck (Turku, Finland) has a system of glass fibers (everStick) that are impregnated with a semi-interpenetrating polymer network (IPN). An IPN network consists of a polymer with 2 or more networks that are not covalently bonded to each other. A semi-IPN network consists only of 1 network and a linear polymer.

The everStick dowel consists of a matrix of a multiphase of bisphenol A diglycidylether methacrylate that is diffused into a linear phase of polymethyl methacrylate (PMMA). A PMMA outer layer surrounds this bundle to increase the adhesive properties of the post. A light-curing bonding resin is then applied to the fiber bundle that was preimpregnated with PMMA and partially dissolves it. A result of this step is the creation of grooves and undercuts that enhance micromechanical bonding. Polymerization results in the monomers forming a cross-link between the cross-linked semi-IPN polymer and phases of the linear polymer.[23] This post system also does not depend on matching drills and provides the best fit of the available post space.

Most fiber reinforced composite posts consist of a resin matrix glass or quartz fibers surrounded by a resin matrix. Quartz fibers have a greater tensile strength than glass fibers. The amount of fibers, their density, and their ability to bond to the resin matrix vary in each system, and consequently, so do their strengths.[24] The resin matrix usually consists of an epoxy resin designed to withstand compressive stresses and absorb stresses in the entire system while the fibers supply tensile strength.[25]

Adhesion to the Post

The ability of the fiber post to resist dislodgement is predicated on the adhesive, the luting material, and the cementation procedure.[26] Adhesive composite cements that are recommended for use have the same elastic modulus as that of the post and dentin. Posts cemented with composite cements exhibit enhanced retention, and the roots are more fracture resistant because of more uniform stress distribution.[27] Failure can also be attributed to inadequate marginal adaptation and subsequent orthograde contamination of the apical terminus.[27] Adhesion between the post, core, and dentin are mediated by the composite resin cement. Despite the many techniques that have been introduced for improving the bond at the post-core interface, breakdown of the bond between the post and resin cement/dentin interface is often the cause of failure.[28] Silane has been recommended to increase bond strength of posts. Fiber-reinforced posts that have highly cross-linked polymers in the matrix do not have functional groups that can chemically interact with silane. The DT Light-Post (Bisco, Schaumburg, IL, USA) has no functional groups that can react with silane, but Style Post (Metalor Dental AG, Bienne, Switzerland) contains hydroxyl (-OH) groups on the surface of the silicate fiber. These groups can form covalent bonds with the silanol group of the silane coupling agent.[29] Airborne particle abrasion with 50-μm aluminum oxide at 2.8 bar (0.28 MPa) pressure for 5 seconds has also been shown to increase surface area and minimize damage.[30]

Self-adhesive cements have been promoted as being simpler and less technique sensitive, but some of them demineralize the dentin, and the depth of resin penetration is not equivalent. In addition, residual acidic monomers may be present, reducing adhesion capabilities.[31] The bonding method of self-adhesive cements involves both chemical interaction and micromechanical interlocking with the substrate. Self-adhesive cements work as dual-cure materials, and the chemical reaction is accomplished by light irradiation. Some studies have indicated lower bond strengths and reduced mechanical properties when the cements are only autocured.[32] This may present a problem, especially in the apical portion, as it is difficult to get light to penetrate to the deepest apical areas.[33] Light scattering in the resin cement is the result of shadowing from tooth structure and the post.[34] Dual-cured resin cements and adhesive systems are usually recommended as combining self-curing and light-curing. Despite the use of 2 initiation systems by some products, adequate light transmission is needed to get light activation and the best results.[35] Translucent glass or quartz fiber posts allow more transmission of light into the root canal space, resulting in increased cure depth.[36] Despite this increased depth of cure, the light transmission is still less than 40% of the incident light.[37] It seems the amine in the base and the peroxide in the catalyst cannot react adequately in the self-cure mode. Although these activation modes are independent, light activation is required to increase the conversion rate.[38,39] If self-etch adhesives are used with self- or dual-cure composite luting materials, there may be an unfavorable reaction between the acidic resin monomers and the tertiary amines that are used in the self-cure systems, resulting in inadequate polymerization and poor bonding. However, if the acidic adhesives are fully cured, this incompatibility would be mitigated. The amount of light and the duration of exposure are critical in reducing the adverse effects of uncured acidic monomers of one-step self-etch adhesives. The mechanical properties of dual-cure adhesives are affected by the duration and amount of light.[39,40]

The needed light energy is affected by the intensity and duration of the light. Aksornmuang and colleagues[41] found that extending the curing time from 10 to 30 seconds increased bond strength by almost 3 times. Because light absorption weakens with increasing cross-sectional distance from the irradiated surface, light at the apical region of a root canal would be greatly reduced.

Adhesion to Intraradicular Dentin

Bonding to intraradicular dentin is erratic. The predentin is a layer that consists of unmineralized organic matrix that lines the deepest pulpal portion and has varying width. The predentin is removed during instrumentation, sodium hypochlorite irrigation, and then by burs used to create the post space. The substrate remaining is mineralized intraradicular dentin. This dentin contains tubules extending from the pulp to the tooth periphery.[42] Intraradicular dentin is similar to coronal dentin, as it contains tubules extending from the pulp to the periphery.[42] The number of tubules decreases toward the apical region, and the ratio between the peritubular and intertubular dentin changes considerably from the apical to the coronal third.[43] Therefore, peritubular dentin infiltration and resin tag formation decrease and intertubular dentin impregnation increases closer to the apex.[44] Theoretically, the increased amount of intertubular dentin present for hybridization should increase bond strength in the apical one-third, but most studies have demonstrated a reduced bond strength in the apical one-third and diminished hybrid layer.[42] The reduced bond strength may possibly be attributed to a negative C-factor.[45]

The variety of material used in an endodontic procedure may also reduce the ability of the clinician to obtain a clean post space. The preparation of the post space with post drills creates a thick smear layer, which consists of debris, sealer, and gutta-percha that reduce the bonding of the post to the intraradicular dentin.[46] The post space should ideally have clean dentinal surfaces to achieve optimal bonding with resin cement.[47] The use of ethylenediaminetetraacetic acid and ultrasonic instrumentation has been suggested to clean the canal, but the bond strength is correlated to the bonding technique used. The use of etch-and-rinse or self-etch creates different results.[48] Methacrylate resins shrink as they polymerize, resulting in shrinkage stress. The shrinkage stress is also related to the cavity configuration (C-factor). The C-factor is the ratio of bonded to unbounded surface areas in a restoration. If the C-factor is high, the stress development may exceed the bond strength of the bonding agent used.[49,50] In a class I cavity, configuration of the C-factor is 5, as there are 5 times more bonded surfaces than unbounded surfaces. The post space can be considered as a deep narrow class I cavity preparation, and because the unbonded surface is small, there is insufficient stress relief by flow.[51] Bouillaguet and colleagues[52] found that C-factors in post spaces can exceed 200.

SUMMARY

The fracture resistance of endodontically treated teeth restored with a fiber post and a composite resin core is better than a tooth restored with a metal post.[53] The wide variety of ceramic crowns used for an anterior restoration require a post and core that do not detract from the aesthetics that can be achieved with these restorations. Thin tissue biotype and a high smile line would benefit from the aesthetic potential of a fiber post and lack of a root discoloration.

REFERENCES

1. Bittner N, Hill T, Randi A. Evaluation of a one-piece milled zirconia post and core with different post-and-core systems: an in vitro study. J Prosthet Dent 2010; 103(6):369–79.
2. Azer SS, Ayash GM, Johnston WM, et al. Effect of esthetic core shades on the final color of IPS Empress all-ceramic crowns. J Prosthet Dent 2006;96(6): 397–401.
3. Zalkind M, Hochman N. Esthetic considerations in restoring endodontically treated teeth with posts. J Prosthet Dent 1998;79(6):702–5.
4. Carossa S, Lombardo S, Pera P, et al. Influence of posts and cores on light transmission through different all-ceramic crowns: spectrophotometric and clinical evaluation. Int J Prosthodont 2001;14(1):9–14.
5. Deger S, Akgüngör G, Caniklioglu B. An alternative method for fabricating a custom-made metal post with a ceramic core. Dent Traumatol 2005;21(3): 179–82.
6. Vichi A, Ferrari M, Davidson CL. Influence of ceramic and cement thickness on the masking of various types of opaque posts. J Prosthet Dent 2000;83(4):412–7.
7. Nakamura T, Saito O, Fuyikawa j, et al. Influence of abutment substrate and ceramic thickness on the colour of heat-pressed ceramic crowns. J Oral Rehabil 2002;29(9):805–9.
8. Michalakis KX, Hirayama H, Sfolkos J, et al. Light transmission of posts and cores used for the anterior region. Int J Periodontics Restorative Dent 2004;24(5): 462–9.
9. de Rouffignac M, de Cooman J. Aesthetic all-porcelain anterior restorations. Pract Periodonics Aesthet Dent 1992;4(8):9–13.
10. Morgano SM, Rodrigues AH, Sabrosa CE. Restoration of endodontically treated teeth. Dent Clin North Am 2004;48(2):397–416.
11. Cheung W. A review of the management of endodontically treated teeth; post, core and the final restoration. J Am Dent Assoc 2005;136(5):611–9.
12. Signore A, Bendicenti S, Kaitsas V, et al. Long-term survival of endodontically treated, maxillary anterior teeth restored with either tapered or parallel-sided glass-fiber posts or full-ceramic crown coverage. J Dent 2009;37(2):115–21.
13. Sorensen JA, Martinoff JT. Edodontically treated teeth as abutments. J Prosthet Dent 1985;53(5):631–6.
14. Theodosopoulou JN, Chochlidakis KM. A systematic review of dowel (post) and core materials. J Prosthodont 2009;18(6):464–72.

15. Peroz I, Blankenstein F, Lange KP, et al. Restoring endodontically treated teeth with post and cores: a review. Quintessence Int 2005;36(9):737–46.
16. Dietschi D, Duc O, Krejci I, et al. Biomechanical considerations for the restoration of endodontically treated teeth: a systematic review of the literature. Part I. Composition and micro and macrostructure alterations. Quintessence Int 2007; 38(9):733–43.
17. Meyenberg KH, Lüthy H, Schärer P. Zirconia posts a new all-ceramic concept for nonvital abutment teeth. J Esthet Dent 1995;7(2):73–80.
18. Stricker EJ, Göhring TN. Influence of different posts and cores on marginal adaptation, fracture resistance and fracture mode of composite resin crowns on human mandibular premolars. An in-vitro study. J Dent 2006;34(5):326–35.
19. Bakke M, Holm B, Jensen BL, et al. Unilateral, isometric bite force in 8–68 year old women and men related top occlusal factors. Scand J Dent Res 1990; 98(2):148–58.
20. Morgano SM, Brackett SE. Foundation restorations in fixed prosthodontics: current knowledge and future needs. J Prosthet Dent 1999;82(6):643–57.
21. Borracchini A, Ferrari M. SEM evaluation of the cement layer thickness after luting two different posts. J Adhes Dent 2005;7(30):235–40.
22. Ferrai M, Vichi A, Mannocci F, et al. Retrospective study of the clinical performance of fiber posts. Am J Dent 2000;13(Spec No):9B–13B.
23. Al-Tayyan MH, Watts DC, Kurer HG, et al. Is a "flexible" glass-bundle dowel system as retentive as a "rigid" quartz fiber dowel system? J Prosthodont 2008;17(7):532–7.
24. Grinding S, Goracci C, Monticelli F, et al. Fatigue resistance and structural characteristics of fiber posts: three point bearing test and SEM evaluation. Dent Mater 2005;21(2):75–82.
25. Seefield F, Wentz HJ, Ludwig K, et al. Resistance to fracture and structural characteristics of different fiber reinforced post systems. Dent Mater 2007;23(3): 265–71.
26. D'Arcangelo C, Zazzeroni S, D'Amario M, et al. Bond strength of three types of fibre-reinforced post systems in various regions of root canals. Int Endod J 2008;41(4):322–8.
27. Zicari F, Couthino E, De Munck JH, et al. Bonding effectiveness and sealing ability of fiber-post bonding. Dent Mater 2008;24(7):967–77.
28. Vichi A, Mannocci F, Mason PN. Retrospective study of clinical performance of fiber posts. Am J Dent 2000;13(Spec No):9B–13B.
29. Kern M, Thompson VP. Sandblasting and silica coating of glass-infiltrated alumina ceramic; volume loss, morphology, and changes in surface composition. J Prosthet Dent 1994;71(5):453–61.
30. Balbosh A, Kjern M. Effect of surface treatment on retention of glass-fiber endodontic posts. J Prosthet Dent 2006;95(3):218–23.
31. Mazzitelli C, Monticelli F. Evaluation of the push-out bond strength of self-adhesive resin to fiber posts. International Dentistry SA 2009;11(6):54–60.
32. Radovic I, Monticelli F, Goracci C, et al. Self adhesive resin cements: a literature review. J Adhes Dent 2008;10(4):251–8.
33. LeBellk AM, Tanner J, Lassila LV, et al. Depth of light-initiated polymerization of glass fiber-reinforced composite in a simulated root canal. Int J Prothodont 2003;16(4):403–8.
34. Faria e Silva AL, Arias VG, Soares LE, et al. Influence of fiber-post translucency on the degree of conversion of a dual-cured resin cement. J Endod 2007;33(3): 303–5.

35. Roberts HW, Leonard DL, Vanderwalle KS, et al. The effect of a translucent post on resin composite depth of cure. Dent Mater 2004;20(7):617–22.
36. Yoldas O, Alaçam T. Microhardness of composites in simulated root canals cured with light transmitting posts and glass-fiber reinforced composite posts. J Endod 2005;31(2):104–6.
37. Teixeira EC, Teixeira FB, Piasick JR, et al. An in vitro assessment of prefabricated fiber post systems. J Am Dent Assoc 2006;137(7):1006–12.
38. Braga RR, Cesar PF, Gonzaga CC. Mechanical properties of resin cements with different activation modes. J Oral Rehabil 2002;29(3):257–62.
39. El-Badrawy WA, El-Mowafy OM. Chemical versus dual curing of resin inlay cements. J Prosthet Dent 1995;73(6):515–24.
40. Tanoue N, Koishi Y, Atsuta M, et al. Properties of dual-curable luting composites polymerized with single and dual curing modes. J Oral Rehabil 2003;30(10): 1015–21.
41. Aksornmuang J, Nakajima M, Panyayong W, et al. Effects of photocuring strategy on bonding of dual-cure one step self-etch adhesive to root canal dentin. Dent Mater J 2009;28(2):133–41.
42. Ferrari M, Mannocci F, Vichi A, et al. Bonding to root canal: structural characteristics of the substrate. Am J Dent 2000;13(5):255–60.
43. Mjor IA, Smith MR, Ferrari M, et al. The structure of dentine in the apical region of human teeth. Int Endod J 2009;34(5):346–53.
44. Mannocci F, Pilecki P, Bertelli E, et al. Density of dentinal tubules affects the tensile strength of root dentin. Dent Mater 2004;20(30):293–6.
45. Breschi L, Mazzoni A, Ferrari M. Adhesion to intra-radicular dentin. In: Ferrari M, Breschi L, Grandini S, editors. Fiber posts and endodontically treated teeth: a compendium of scientific and clinical perspectives. Wendywood (SA): Modern Dentistry Media; 2008. p. 15–37.
46. Goracci C, Sadek FT, Fabianelli A, et al. Evaluation of the adhesion of fiber posts to intradicular dentin. Oper Dent 2005;30(5):627–35.
47. Boone KJ, Murchison DF, Schindler WG, et al. Post retention: the effect of sequence of post preparation, cementation time, and different sealers. J Endod 2001;27(12):768–71.
48. Coniglio I, Magni E, Goracci C, et al. Post space cleaning using a new nickel titanium endodontic drill combined with different cleaning regimens. J Endod 2008; 34(1):83–6.
49. Feilzer AJ, DeGee AJ, Davidson CL. Setting stress in composite resin in relation to configuration of the restoration. J Dent Res 1987;66(11):1636–9.
50. Tay FR, Loushine RJ, Lambrechts P, et al. Geometric factors affecting dentin bonding in root canals: a theoretical modeling approach. J Endod 2005;31(8): 584–9.
51. Goracci C, Fabianelli A, Sadek FT, et al. The contribution of friction to the dislocation resistance of bonded fiber posts. J Endod 2005;31(8):608–12.
52. Bouillaguet S, Troesch S, Wataha JC, et al. Microtensile bond strength between adhesive cements and root canal dentin. Dent Mater 2003;19(3):199–205.
53. Hayashi M, Sugeta A, Takahashi Y, et al. Static and fatigue fracture resistances of pulpless teeth restored with post-cores. Dent Mater 2008;24(9):1178–86.

Index

Note: Page numbers of article titles are in **boldface** type.

A

Acrylic resin veneering technique, 354
Adhesives, and cements, for all-ceramic restorations, **311–332**
Airborne particle abrasion, for improved resin bonding, 325–326
All-ceramic materials, bonding interface of, 322–327
All-ceramic restorations, cements and adhesives for, **311–332**
All-ceramic systems, bonding strategies for, 323
    laboratory and clinical performance of, **333–352**
    laboratory performance of, 344–346
    mechanical properties of, 334
    new concepts for, 346
American Academy of Cosmetic Dentistry, standard series of photographs, 213
Axial inclination, 202

B

Bite wings, 198
Bleaching, adverse effects on enamel, 257–258
    adverse effects on gingiva, 258
    adverse effects on pulp, 258
    adverse effects on restorative materials, 259
    local adverse effects associated with, 257–259
    of single discolored tooth. See *Tooth (Teeth), single discolored.*
    roles of dental professionals in, 260
    safety concerns with no involvement of dental professionals, 258–259
    safety controversies in, **255–263**
    tooth sensitivity and, 258–259
    vital, case selection for, minimizing risks and side effects of, 242–243, 244
        in-office, light-assisted, appeal of, 241
            variability associated with, 244–250
            variability in shade evaluation and color-measuring instruments, 245, 248
            variability with different light sources, 245–249
            variability with different lights and bleaching formula interactions, 249–250
            variability with UV light and dentinal absorption, 250
        professional supervision for, 242
        setting expectations of treatment time, 243–244
        with adjunct light, **241–253**
Bridge, resin-bonded, 291–292
Buccal view, 197, 198

C

Canine substitution, bracket placement in, 285
Carbamide peroxide, 232, 255

Dent Clin N Am 55 (2011) 411–417
doi:10.1016/S0011-8532(11)00044-9
0011-8532/11/$ – see front matter © 2011 Elsevier Inc. All rights reserved.

dental.theclinics.com

Moving?

Make sure your subscription moves with you!

To notify us of your new address, find your **Clinics Account Number** (located on your mailing label above your name), and contact customer service at:

Email: journalscustomerservice-usa@elsevier.com

800-654-2452 (subscribers in the U.S. & Canada)
314-447-8871 (subscribers outside of the U.S. & Canada)

Fax number: 314-447-8029

Elsevier Health Sciences Division
Subscription Customer Service
3251 Riverport Lane
Maryland Heights, MO 63043

*To ensure uninterrupted delivery of your subscription, please notify us at least 4 weeks in advance of move.

Printed and bound by CPI Group (UK) Ltd, Croydon, CR0 4YY

03/10/2024

01040459-0006